THE APPLE CIDER VINEGAR CURE

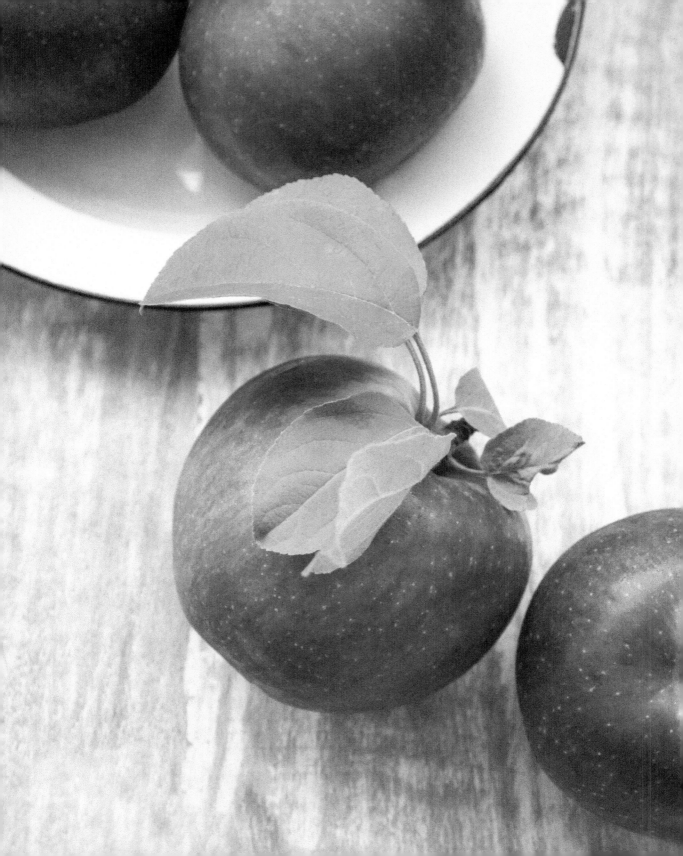

The
APPLE CIDER VINEGAR CURE

Essential Recipes and Remedies to Heal Your Body Inside and Out

MADELINE GIVEN, NC

SONOMA
PRESS

DEDICATION

For David—very much so.

For general information on our other products and services or to obtain technical support, please contact our Customer Care Department within the United States at (866) 744-2665, or outside the United States at (510) 253-0500.

Sonoma Press publishes its books in a variety of electronic and print formats. Some content that appears in print may not be available in electronic books, and vice versa.

TRADEMARKS: Sonoma Press and the Sonoma Press logo are trademarks or registered trademarks of Callisto Media Inc. and/or its affiliates, in the United States and other countries, and may not be used without written permission. All other trademarks are the property of their respective owners. Sonoma Press is not associated with any product or vendor mentioned in this book.

Illustrations © 2015 by Tom Bingham

Front cover photography © (clockwise from top left) Stocksy/Harald Walker; Stockfood/Jennifer Blume; Stockfood/Victoria Firmston; Stockfood/Ian Garlick; Suzanne Clements; Stocksy/Trinette Reed. Back cover photography © (clockwise from top left) Stocksy/Cameron Whitman; Shutterstock/Potapov Alexander; Stocksy/Todor Vassilev; and Suzanne Clements. Interior photography © Stockfood/Jennifer Blume, p.2; Stocksy/Jeff Wasserman, p.5, 86; Stocksy/Trinette Reed, p.5, 47; Stocksy/Sara Remington, p.5, 117; Stocksy/Jeff Wasserman, p.10; Suzanne Clements, p.12; Shannon Oslick, p.17; Shutterstock/CatchaSnap, p.17; Stocksy/David Smart, p.20; Stockfood/Food Experts Group, p.30; Suzanne Clements, p.35; Stocksy/Helen Rushbrook, p.40; Stocksy/Trinette Reed, p.42; Shutterstock/matka_Wariatka, p.53; Stocksy/Jon Attaway, p.57; Shutterstock/John Goldstein, p.63; Stockfood/Valerie Jensen, p.64; Stocksy/Pavel Gramatikov, p.67; Shutterstock/joannawnuk, p.79; Stocksy/Ina Peters, p.81; Stocksy/Aleksandar Novoselski, p.83; Stocksy/Jeff Wasserman, p.86; Stockfood/Victoria Firmston, p.88; Stockfood/Bernhard Winkelmann, p.95; Stocksy/Ina Peters, p.100; Stockfood/Ian Garlick, p.107; Stocksy/Cameron Whitman, p.108; Stockfood/Alicia Manas Aldaya, p.122; Stockfood/Jo Kirchherr, p.127; Stockfood/Tate Carlson, p.132; Stockfood/Emel Ernalbant, p.136; Stockfood/Gräfe & Unzer Verlag/Coco Lang, p.143; Stocksy/Darren Muir, p.148; Stocksy/Noemi Hauser, p.153; Stockfood/Leigh Beisch, p.156; Stockfood/Greg Rannells Photography, p.164; Stockfood/Ian Garlick, p.171; Stocksy/Laura Adani, p.178; Stocksy/Federica Di Marcello, p.185; Gantes.co, p.216

ISBN: Print 978-1-942411-27-7
eBook 978-1-942411-28-4

QUICK-START GUIDE

Whether you're an apple cider vinegar veteran or you've just picked up your first bottle at the grocery store, we're confident that, in the pages that follow, you'll find new and intriguing ways to use this tried-and-true natural liquid. If you want to reap the benefits of apple cider vinegar right away, we invite you to skip ahead to any of the following parts of the book that immediately draw you in.

Read up on the history of apple cider vinegar to learn how this timeless tonic has been used for centuries in folklore medicine. *See page 13.*

Try out simple ailment remedies that use basic applications of this therapeutic liquid. *See page 26.*

Learn to make apple cider vinegar at home, with tips on everything from apple selection to avoiding mistakes even the pros make. *See page 31.*

Create your own healing remedies and effective body and hair care treatments. *See page 41.*

Discover new recipes that use apple cider vinegar in savory and sweet dishes—keeping you nourished at every meal. *See page 87.*

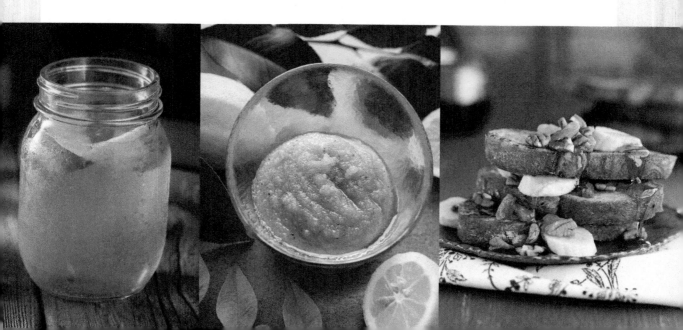

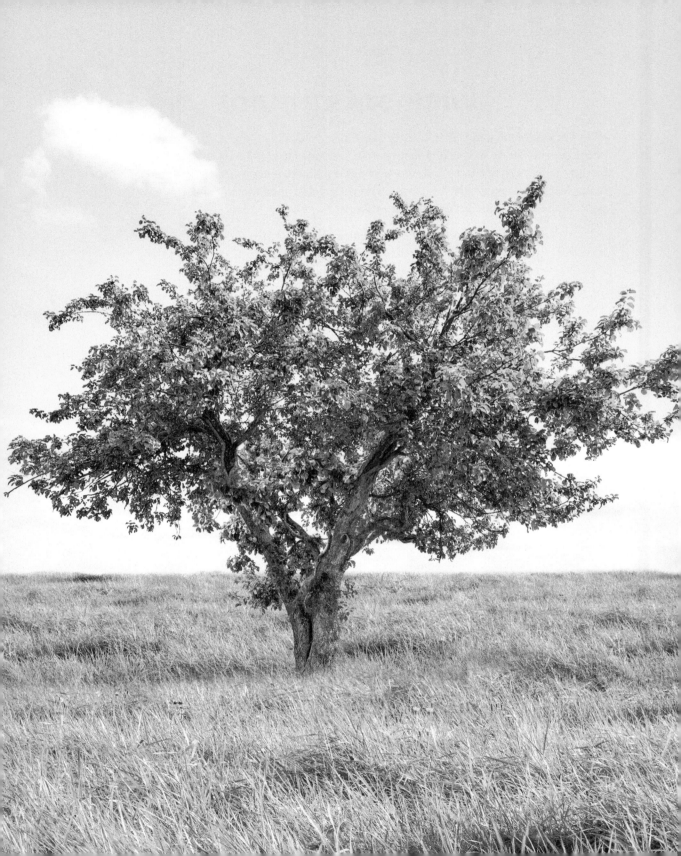

CONTENTS

Introduction • 8

EXPLORING APPLE CIDER VINEGAR

The Rebirth of Vinegar • 13

A Tablespoon a Day • 21

Homemade Apple Cider Vinegar • 31

REMEDIES

Body & Hair Care • 43

Common Ailments • 65

RECIPES

Drinks & Smoothies • 89

Breakfast • 109

Condiments & Sides • 123

Soups & Salads • 137

Entrées • 157

Desserts • 179

Appendix A: Conversion Tables • 199

Appendix B: The Dirty Dozen
& The Clean Fifteen • 200

Resources • 201

References • 202

Remedy & Recipe Index • 203

Index • 205

About the Author • 216

INTRODUCTION

Discovering Your Own Irreplaceable Uses
for Apple Cider Vinegar

A SIMPLE INTERNET SEARCH for "apple cider vinegar" will turn up quite a mix of results—from enthusiastic celebrity claims for instantaneous weight loss to traditional recipes for pickling vegetables. Apple cider vinegar has an initial pungent odor, astringent on the nose and bursting with ripe acids. The taste is bitter yet refreshingly sweet, and will instantly energize the gut. When unfiltered, the amber liquid appears cloudy. What exactly is this humble elixir all about?

While we recognize healthful vinegars as one of the micro-trends of the current decade, vinegar residues found in urns from ancient Egypt have been traced back to 3000 BC! And it's been reported that Hippocrates, widely respected as the father of herbal medicine, was prescribing a mixture of apple cider vinegar and honey for coughs and colds in Greece as early as 400 BC.

As a holistic nutritionist, I've recommended apple cider vinegar to many of my clients for numerous afflictions, but most often for an out-of-whack digestive tract. When I hear reports of symptoms like bloating, indigestion, and heartburn, I know the culprit will usually be a deficiency of stomach acid. The less-than-nourishing standard American diet of processed foods only serves to make our body's many systems more acidic and disease-prone. Ironically, this way of eating also leads to an unfortunate lowering of acid in one of the main organs that actually requires acid for proper function: the stomach. Rather than popping an antacid pill, I recommend mixing a tablespoon of raw apple cider vinegar in a glass of water when symptoms first appear. Voilà! Be at peace with your stomach.

I use apple cider vinegar in my daily regimen, both topically and internally. My favorite facial toners combine apple cider vinegar with one or two essential oils and some witch hazel for a reviving skin treatment morning or night. When diluted with water and a little lemon juice and honey, it's the perfect wake-up beverage for my stomach before breakfast, setting the stage for proper digestion through-out the day. Many mornings, I find it even more invigorating than a cup of coffee.

Are you ready to discover your own irreplaceable uses for this multi-purpose liquid?

Part One: Exploring Apple Cider Vinegar walks you through the rebirth of this historical tonic and details the ways a mere tablespoon a day can make a difference in your life. You'll also learn how to make your own batch at home. It's easier than you think—all you need are some apple scraps, water, and a little honey or sugar.

Once you've taken a stab at making your own apple cider vinegar, we don't want you to waste any time before using it. Jump right in to **Part Two: Remedies**, where you'll find over 40 unique remedies for body and hair care, plus relief for common ailments.

Finally, **Part Three: Recipes** offers 75 delicious and simple recipes for every meal of the day as you explore ways to use apple cider vinegar in your kitchen. Let's get started!

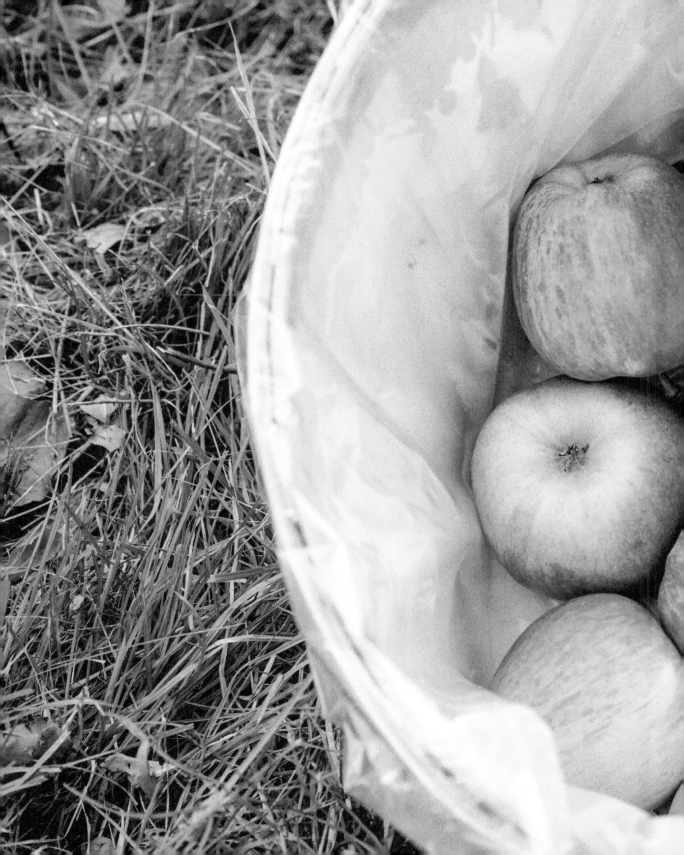

Exploring Apple Cider Vinegar

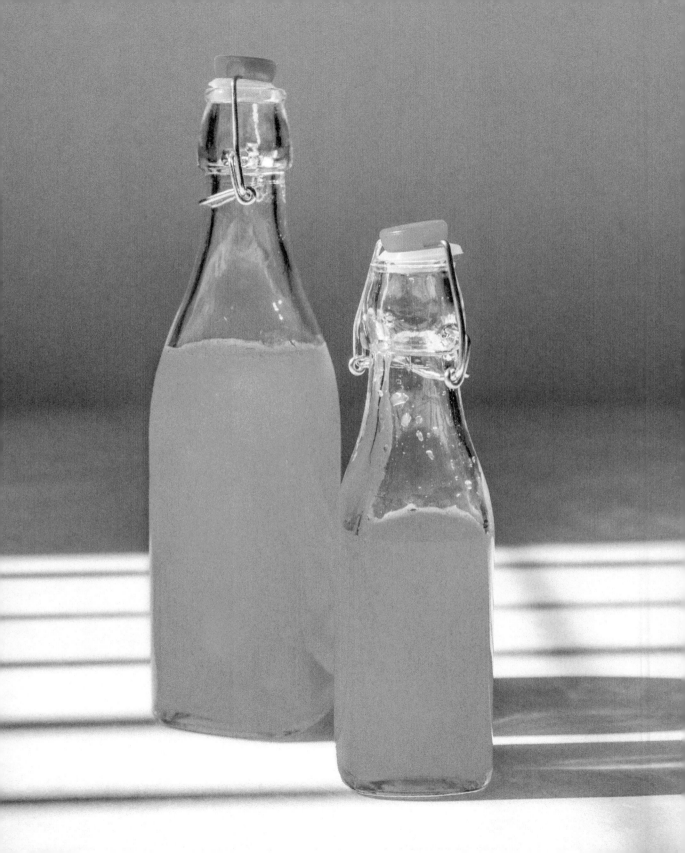

Chapter One

THE REBIRTH OF VINEGAR

GIVE YOUR GLASS BOTTLE of apple cider vinegar a good shake. Is it raw and cloudy? Filtered and translucent?

Let's take an in-depth look at this historical, fermented superfood that has been experiencing a resurgence in popularity and nontraditional uses in the past decade. While scientific studies of apple cider vinegar are few and far between, stories from the past and anecdotal evidence are in large supply. Once you explore its use as part of a healthy lifestyle, apple cider vinegar will quickly find a permanent place in your kitchen.

WHAT IS VINEGAR?

One ripe apple contains all the building blocks of apple cider vinegar—it just needs a little coaching to undergo transformation from sweet fruit to tart vinegar. In its most basic definition, *vinegar is a sour-tasting liquid containing acetic acid and water, made through a two-step fermentation process*. Traditional vinegar simply requires raw materials that contain sugar or starch, such as grapes, apples, rice, or potatoes. The fermentation process starts when the natural sugars are left to change into alcohol over several weeks. When acetic acid bacteria, which are naturally present everywhere in the environment, begin to oxygenate the mix, the alcohol converts to acetic acid.

While there is a definitive science to the process of creating vinegar, it's possible to end up with a motley batch accidentally: an opened bottle of wine forgotten for months on a shelf; fruit scraps or juice left in a pantry now ripe with acidic potency. The smell may cause you to wrinkle your nose, but don't turn away just yet. There are hundreds of potential uses to explore.

For years, vinegar has been used in every room of the house and for almost every part of the body. It's commonly used in the kitchen to pickle fruits and vegetables, and to prepare dressings and condiments. Its antibacterial strength is touted as an effective home cleaner for everything from floor to ceiling. And it has even been suggested that the therapeutic capacities of vinegar include lowering blood pressure and reducing the effects of type 2 diabetes.

MAKING APPLE CIDER VINEGAR

Arguably, apple cider vinegar has been the most popular vinegar in the United States since the eighteenth century. There are several methods used today to produce vinegar, but the traditional method consists of apples, water, air, and time.

During the first part of the fermentation process, the simple sugars in the raw materials are changed to alcohol by yeasts also naturally present in the fruit. This alcohol is then oxidized into acetic acid by acetic acid bacteria during the second phase. The full maturation process can take anywhere from one week to several months, or longer.

UNFILTERED VERSUS FILTERED

While apple cider vinegar is being made, the acetic acid bacteria culture can be either left untouched to float on top or submerged into the liquid. Traditionally, the culture was left to rest, requiring more time for the fermentation medium to reach the entire batch of liquid. To speed the process, most commercial manufacturers oxygenate the liquid by rapidly submerging the culture into the liquid, thus speeding up the fermentation process.

When left untouched to ferment naturally, a slimy glob of yeast and acetic acid bacteria will form at the surface of the liquid. This substance is known as the "mother" of the vinegar. At this point, the science becomes both fascinating and gross at the same time: Microscopic vinegar eels (*Turbatrix aceti*) form to feed on the mother if the liquid is left for a longer fermentation period and the mother is not removed before bottling. Vinegar eels are harmless, nonparasitic nematodes and their health benefits far outweigh any qualms you have about consuming them. However, some manufacturers choose to remove these organisms before bottling. If processed and removed, the apple cider vinegar is considered filtered.

Many health advocates argue that the mother should be left in the vinegar when stored, because it retains numerous health benefits. If you choose to purchase unfiltered apple cider vinegar, it should appear muddy and you should be able to see bits of the mother floating around. This means you'll be getting the maximum amount of enzymes, health-promoting organic acids, and living, beneficial bacteria that apple cider vinegar has to offer.

RAW VERSUS PASTEURIZED

When you purchase a raw food product, it typically means that the product is closest to its most natural form and state. Purchasing raw apple cider vinegar means you should get an unrefined, unpasteurized, and unfiltered vinegar that was not subjected to any artificial processes, nor had anything added. No naturally occurring enzymes or bioactive compounds have been harmed in raw vinegar.

On the other hand, pasteurized vinegar has undergone a partial sterilization process involving high heat or irradiation to kill any harmful bacteria that may cause it to spoil or promote disease.

If you purchase raw and unpasteurized apple cider vinegar, buy a trusted brand from a trusted store. It's crucial that the manufacturer uses the best and safest practices as well as sterile equipment when handling the unpasteurized product, to avoid contamination by disease-causing microorganisms. In the same vein, if you purchase unpasteurized apples or apple juice to make your own vinegar, be sure to buy fresh-pressed apple cider and organically grown apples from a local, well-known farm.

WHY MAKE YOUR OWN VINEGAR?

Making your own apple cider vinegar may sound like a daunting, time-consuming task, but the hands-on time is extremely small and yields an incredible payout. It's often not even necessary to purchase special ingredients for a homemade batch of apple cider vinegar—you probably have the items in your pantry already.

While the average grocery store chain most likely carries pasteurized apple cider vinegar at an affordable price, to try this medicinal tonic in its purest and rawest form, you may end up paying a pretty penny, depending on the grocer you frequent. Thankfully, making your own raw vinegar is extraordinarily cost effective, especially if you're able to use apple scraps, peels, and cores left over from snack time or an apple-filled recipe. The at-home method is also the best way to guarantee you're getting additive-free, unrefined vinegar and all the health advantages that come with it (see page 31 to learn how to make your own).

Experimenting with making your own vinegar will give you the confidence and contentment that comes from successfully creating something from scratch with your own two hands. It can easily be crafted into a fun and educational food science experiment for both kids and adults. And, once you've accomplished the fermentation of your first batch, you won't want to see it go to waste. All your patience and diligent work will encourage you to use this versatile product daily for your body *and* home.

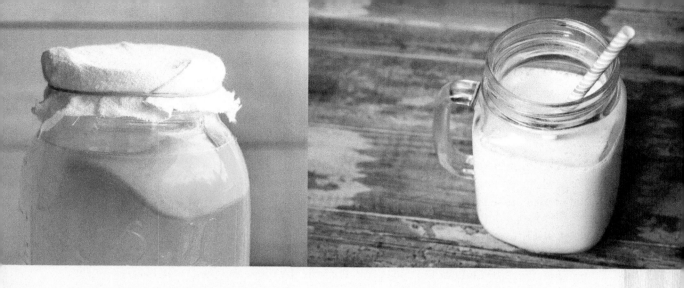

On Trend: Fermentation

Even though apple cider vinegar has been around for several millennia, there's no denying it has seen a recent rebirth in our lifetime. Fermented beverages are on point right now, especially in the healthful food world of organic juice bars and farm-to-table restaurants. They all boast a tastiness that is bursting with beneficial probiotic bacteria. Many fermented drinks have experienced a resurgence in popularity lately, even though their origins date back many centuries and emanate from all over the world, including:

KOMBUCHA: This fermented tea begins with a slimy mother similar to that of apple cider vinegar. This starter is called a SCOBY, which stands for *symbiotic colony of bacteria and yeast.* Once combined with sweetened tea, kombucha is formed in as little as one week of fermentation. Per ancient folklore, kombucha has been around since the Chinese Qin dynasty of the third century BC, and its reputation for vitality spread via trade routes throughout Asia and Eastern Europe. It didn't enter mainstream American markets until the 1960s, where it received the nickname "hippie tea" by its home brewers. Now anyone can purchase a bottle of kombucha at their local Whole Foods Market for $3 to $8.

KEFIR: Yogurt-like in consistency, kefir is a sour-tasting drink traditionally made from cow's milk fermented with a specific bacteria-yeast culture referred to as "grains." It is said to have originated in the Caucasus Mountains in Eastern Europe around 3000 BC. If you don't consume dairy, try water kefir, which starts with similarly cultured "grains" and a sugar-water mixture. The bacteria consume most of the sugar, leaving behind a slightly effervescent and not-too-sweet beverage full of many unique strains of probiotic bacteria.

KVASS: Also rooted deeply in Eastern European history (mainly Russia), kvass is another fermented drink, low in alcohol, traditionally made from rye bread and flavored with produce ranging from sweet strawberries to tangy mint. It can be added to soups and stews to aid in proper digestion and provide a healthy dose of friendly bacteria and enzymes. Compared with the other fermented drinks listed, kvass has a more malted taste somewhat similar to beer. Kvass can also be made from beets, creating a medicinal tonic with powerful liver- and gallbladder-cleansing properties.

VINEGAR THROUGHOUT HISTORY

The word vinegar stems from the French *vin aigre*, which literally means sour wine. Different varieties of vinegar hail from different countries: balsamic vinegar originally came from Italy; Champagne vinegar from France; rice vinegar from China and Japan. Apple cider vinegar, however, has roots all over the world.

Apple cider vinegar's history is rife with old wives' tales and communal stories passed down orally through generations.

In Medicine

Medicinal uses for vinegar developed and became more widely known and practiced throughout the Old World. Possibly the most accepted folklore about apple cider vinegar concerns Hippocrates and his medicinal prescription of the tonic to help heal wounds around 420 BC.

Chinese physician Sung Tse is credited with creating forensic medicine in the tenth century as we've come to know it today. He picked up on the antibacterial effects of vinegar early on and is known for being one of the first physicians to promote hand washing with sulfur and vinegar to avoid infection during surgery.

In the last several centuries, US medical practitioners have documented a wide variety of apple cider vinegar's medicinal uses, including for:

- Allergies and congestion
- Candida yeast overgrowth
- Corns, calluses, and warts
- Croup
- Dropsy
- Granular myringitis
- Heartburn
- High cholesterol
- Hypertension
- Hypoglycemia
- Kidney stones
- Oral bacteria
- Poison ivy and poison oak
- Stomachaches

In History and Culture

Romanticized tales of vinegar's power are scattered throughout history. Hannibal of Carthage (c. 200 BC) is said to have dissolved entire boulders with fire and vinegar when a landslide threatened to hold back his troops as they traipsed through the Alps.

Cleopatra (c. 50 BC) won a bet against Marc Antony when she claimed she could spend 10 million sesterces (a small fortune) on one meal. She then had her servants bring her a single goblet of vinegar, into which she tossed one of her pearl earrings. Legend has it that the pearl dissolved in the vinegar and she swallowed her homemade love potion before a dumbfounded Marc Antony. When classicist Prudence Jones of Montclair State University in New Jersey set out to prove the plausibility of this tale of antiquity, she used a 5 percent solution of acetic acid and found it takes 24 to 36 hours to completely dissolve a pearl weighing around 1 gram (0.035 ounce)—and it is drinkable.

In Food

According to our limited oral history of this elixir, the Babylonians were the first to use vinegar around 5000 BC. Legend has it that a royal attendant first came across "accidental wine" that had fermented from neglected grape juice. Not surprising, the next thing he noticed was that some of it had begun to ferment further and turn into vinegar. This discovery was the start of vinegar's popular use as a food and pickling agent.

Scientists discovered what appeared to be vinegar residues in ancient Egyptian urns dating back to about 3000 BC, while the first written history of vinegar didn't appear until approximately 1200 BC in ancient Chinese texts.

The first vinegar fans were not necessarily on a mission to find a miracle cure-all; most just loved it for its practicality in the pantry. Preserving food by pickling is an ancient art. Many archaeologists have labeled Mesopotamia as the first-ever pickling hub, prior to 2400 BC. Shortly thereafter, pickling spread to India, where they first experimented with the traditional dill pickle's crucial piece of produce: the cucumber.

Preserving foods with vinegar was a godsend to early troops as well—Napoleon reportedly offered a reward to anyone who came up with a way to feed his armies cucumbers (his personal favorite vegetable) when they were out in the field long-term.

In the eighteenth and nineteenth centuries in the United States, farm workers created a drink made from cider vinegar, water, honey, and ginger, which they called a switchel. Looking back, it appears that this was the first "energy drink" offered to fatigued laborers in America, only adding to apple cider vinegar's popularity and many uses.

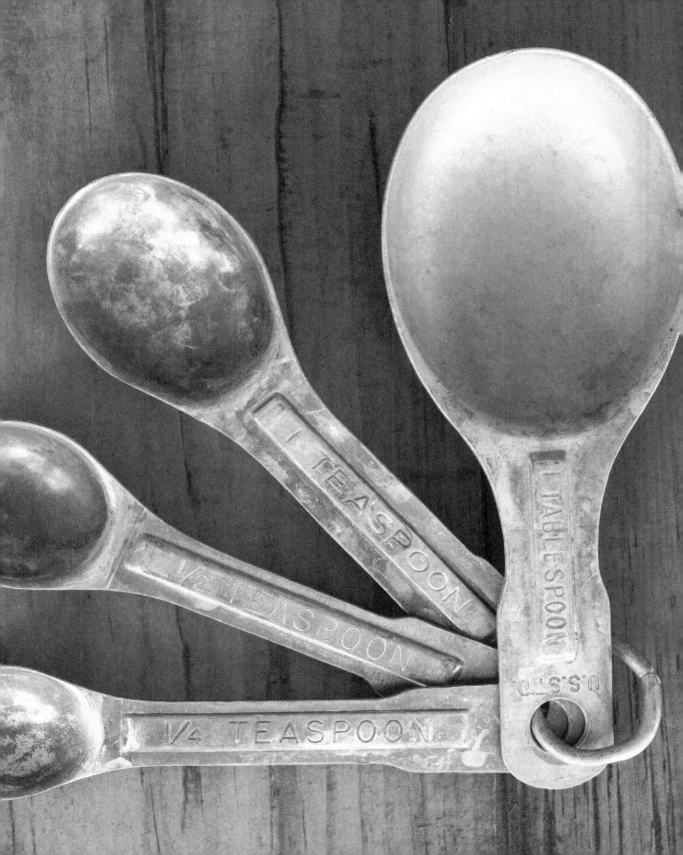

Chapter Two

A TABLESPOON A DAY

WE'VE ALL HEARD THE OLD ADAGE, "An apple a day keeps the doctor away." But could the same be true for just a tablespoon of apple cider vinegar? We now know it's a multipurpose workhorse with a versatile array of applications, and we've learned some of the history behind the hype. In this chapter, we'll explore apple cider vinegar's scientific makeup and discuss ways this restorative tonic can safely be used to improve your health and upgrade your beauty routine.

A TIMELESS TONIC

People have been using apple cider vinegar for hundreds of years. When the ancient Romans imported a variety of foods from the countries they conquered, they were quick to realize the items wouldn't survive the journey unless they preserved them in vinegar. And Christopher Columbus is said to have brought barrels of this health tonic on his ships to prevent scurvy in his crew.

If you take a quick look online, you'll find hundreds of apple cider vinegar enthusiasts claiming they've treated everything from obesity to dandruff with this purportedly magical tonic. And despite a slight lingering skepticism from health professionals and scientists, apple cider vinegar is still being pushed by the masses as the perfect remedy for countless ailments.

While this book focuses on presenting the anecdotal pros and cons so you can discern for yourself where apple cider vinegar might fit into your lifestyle, there is also a handful of science-backed claims to report. Recently there have been several studies done with apple cider vinegar yielding promising research on cholesterol levels, weight loss, and type 2 diabetes. One such study indicated that apple cider vinegar improved the serum lipid profile in both healthy and diabetic rats by decreasing their serum triglyceride levels and LDL-cholesterol while increasing their serum HDL-cholesterol—great news for those with diabetic complications.

There are also a number of researchers who agree that ingesting vinegar may decrease the glycemic effect of a meal through feelings of satiation, so one would potentially consume less food in general. Again, this has only been officially tested in rats fed vinegar extract, the majority of which ended up having lower body weight, fasting postprandial glucose, and plasma insulin concentrations than the controls.

WHAT DOES SCIENCE HAVE TO SAY?

The major chemical component of vinegar is acetic acid, or ethanoic acid (CH_3COOH). Most vinegars are composed of 5 percent acetic acid and 95 percent water. This volatile organic acid is formed in the fermentation process through a group of bacteria called acetic acid bacteria (AAB) that are part of the family Acetobacteriaceae. Unique species of AAB have been isolated from different kinds of vinegars. For example, apple cider vinegar contains *Acetobacter aceti*, *A. intermedius*,

A. pasteurianus, Gluconacetobacter europaeus, G. hansenii, and *G. xylinus.* All these bacteria require oxygen to flourish and carry the fermentation process on to fruition.

Once the oxidation process begins to work on the sugar in the apples and the alcohol in the cider, the AAB produce an array of organic acids that are unique to each type of vinegar. This is the good stuff; vinegar's nutritious reputation is due in large part to these volatile compounds. Apple cider vinegar, in particular, can contain a lengthy list of organic acids, including but not limited to acetic, citric, formic, lactic, malic, and succinic acids.

The acetic acid in apple cider vinegar is able to pass into cell membranes of microorganisms, which is a fancy way of saying that apple cider vinegar possesses antibacterial properties. The effects of organic acids were studied in 1998, and acetic acid was found to be the most effective at killing the dreaded *Escherichia coli* (*E. coli*) bacteria.

In the end, however, vinegar is not only low in calories, but low in both macro- and micronutrients as well. One cup of vinegar is typically 98.8 percent water and contains around 30 to 50 calories, no fat or protein, and only a few grams of carbohydrates. While some tout its high potassium and mineral content, the actual amount of these micronutrients is quite miniscule when the small 1-cup serving size is taken into consideration; potassium is the most present at only 240 milligrams per cup.

So if the vitamin and nutrient claims are not all they are cracked up to be, where does apple cider vinegar get its power? New research suggests that while vinegar isn't boasting its own impressive nutrient profile, its acetic acid can increase our bodies' absorption of important nutrients from other foods we consume.

Scientists are also currently studying beneficial compounds in plants called phytochemicals. These natural and restorative plant remedies are often overlooked in a world where pharmaceutical drugs seem to reign. However, studies have begun to show how plant-based products made from fruits and vegetables—like our very own apple cider vinegar—address the root of the disease, while synthetic drugs often mask the problem, offering only symptomatic relief.

Vinegars are rich in polyphenols, a group of phytochemicals synthesized by plants to defend against their own oxidative stress. When humans consume these polyphenols, they enhance their antioxidant protection because they are, essentially, consuming the immune systems of the plants. These polyphenols are currently being studied for their possible link to cancer prevention.

RESTORATIVE INSIDE AND OUT

If you have an interest in your gut and what's good for it, this apple cider vinegar odyssey could be a health goldmine for you. Model and television host Heidi Klum mixes a couple tablespoons of apple cider vinegar with a full glass of water before meals because she feels it cleanses her system and makes her body internally more alkaline. But the age-old elixir has plenty of advantages for your body's exterior as well. Actress Scarlett Johansson uses apple cider vinegar as her "$5 beauty treatment" to restore her skin's natural pH levels and accentuate her glow.

Vinegar Precautions

Because of its acidic nature, vinegar could burn the oral cavity, esophagus, and upper opening of the stomach when taken orally. Chronic inflammation of these sensitive tissues is a cancer risk. **ALWAYS PROPERLY DILUTE VINEGAR BEFORE INGESTING:**

The suggested dilution is 1 to 2 tablespoons of vinegar per 8 ounces of water or juice.

We've sung its praises for pages now, but where should we tap the brakes with apple cider vinegar?

TEETH: Vinegar's harsh acetic acid can damage or soften tooth enamel if not diluted properly or if left to linger too long on these delicate areas. Always rinse your mouth with water after consuming apple cider vinegar. And because vinegar can soften tooth enamel, it's best to wait 1 hour after use before brushing your teeth, to avoid damaging sensitive enamel with tough bristles.

ALLERGIC REACTION OR IRRITATION: To prevent potential allergic reactions or skin irritation, always test any topical tinctures that include apple cider vinegar on a small part of your skin before putting it on a larger portion of your skin.

BURNS: Avoid apple cider vinegar tablets or capsules, since they could become stuck in your throat and cause esophageal burns.

STOMACH: If apple cider vinegar does not agree with your stomach, discontinue its use.

PREGNANCY AND NURSING: Not enough studies have been done concerning pregnant or nursing women and apple cider vinegar consumption. If pregnant or nursing, we encourage you to do your own research and proceed with common sense and caution.

PRESCRIPTION MEDICINE INTERACTIONS: If you are currently taking any other supplements or prescription medications, always consult your doctor before adding apple cider vinegar to your daily health regimen.

Arthritis Relief

Apple cider vinegar benefits are also reported as more than just skin deep—anecdotal evidence points toward its ability to fight, if not cure, arthritis, which is an inflammation of the joints. A nurse named Margaret Hills first experimented with apple cider vinegar's effect on arthritis in 1961; she believed that arthritis was caused by an overabundance of acid crystals lodged in the joints, causing pain and stiffness. Ergo, the thought process was to get rid of the acidic environment, thereby getting rid of the arthritis. And while vinegar is an acid by nature, the overall effect of a homemade tonic like apple cider vinegar and honey is actually alkalizing to the body once it hits the stomach, making it the perfect natural remedy to try in this case.

Manage Morning Sickness

While we've previously cautioned pregnant and nursing women to check with their doctors before using apple cider vinegar therapeutically, those who have done so suggest that it can help assuage morning sickness associated with pregnancy, as well as a general lack of appetite. When stomach acid is too low or too high, apple cider vinegar can step in to help neutralize it, especially when mixed with a stomach-soothing tea, such as ginger or chamomile.

Clear Acne

Because apple cider vinegar promotes alkalinity in the body, estheticians and skin care specialists are beginning to recommend drinking vinegar concoctions as a recipe for clearing acne-cluttered skin. The trend in the beauty world right now is to add beauty foods to the diet rather than relying solely on topical creams and applications. Apple cider vinegar fits the bill for both.

Smile and Breathe Fresh

Some progressive dentists recommend a diluted apple cider vinegar mouthwash for a more organic way to whiten teeth and kill germs responsible for bad breath. Simply swish two parts water to one part apple cider vinegar in your mouth up to 1 minute and rinse your teeth thoroughly with water afterward.

A VERSATILE LIQUID

While apple cider vinegar is not a panacea for every ache and pain, it can still be a strong component of a healthy lifestyle. We encourage you to continue to research the potential benefits of apple cider vinegar and test out various remedies to see what works for your body. Which of the following simple remedies do you think you'll try first?

AILMENT	APPLE CIDER VINEGAR	OTHER LIQUID	OTHER INGREDIENT	APPLICATION
Acne	2 tablespoons	NA	2 to 3 tablespoons baking soda	Apply to face as a mask. Leave on 10 to 20 minutes until dry. Rinse off with cool water. Repeat once a week.
Allergies	1 tablespoon	1 tablespoon freshly squeezed lemon juice	½ tablespoon raw honey	Mix well. Drink three times a day during allergy season.
Athlete's foot	1 part	1 part lukewarm water	NA	Soak feet in 50/50 solution twice daily.
Bald spots	1 teaspoon	NA	Dash cayenne	Massage onto bald spot once a week to stimulate growth.
Blood sugar regulation	2 tablespoons	1 cup water	1 tablespoon raw honey	Drink mixture before bed to control waking glucose levels.
Candida overgrowth	1 teaspoon	1 cup water	NA	Drink once a day.
Cellulite	3 parts	NA	1 part organic olive oil	Combine and firmly massage into trouble area daily.
Congestion	1 part	1 part water	NA	Heat the mixture and inhale the steam.
Dandruff	2 to 3 tablespoons	Sponge full of water	NA	Sponge vinegar evenly onto scalp before shampooing.
Detox cleansing	1 tablespoon	1 cup organic green tea	Raw honey to taste	Prepare tea with honey. Allow tea to cool before mixing in vinegar and sipping.
Eczema	½ cup	½ cup water	2 tablespoons evening primrose oil	Combine vinegar with water and pat affected areas using a soft cloth. Follow with a light layer of evening primrose oil.
Fatigue	2 teaspoons	1 cup water	2 teaspoons raw honey	Mix well. Drink when you need an energy boost.
Heartburn	1 teaspoon	1 cup water	NA	Drink after each meal.
Jellyfish stings	1 tablespoon	NA	NA	Use straight vinegar on infected area, or dilute as needed.
Joint pain	1 cup	Bathtub of warm water	1 cup Epsom salts	Combine mixture in bathtub and soak up to 30 minutes.

AILMENT	APPLE CIDER VINEGAR	OTHER LIQUID	OTHER INGREDIENT	APPLICATION
Large pores	1 teaspoon	2 teaspoons water	1 drop lavender essential oil	Combine and wipe over face with an organic cotton pad. No need to rinse.
Leg cramps	2 teaspoons	1 cup water	1 to 2 teaspoons raw honey	Drink three times a day to relieve cramping.
Lice	1 (15-ounce) bottle	1 to 2 cups melted coconut oil	10 drops tea tree essential oil	Completely rinse hair with vinegar. Mix oils and rub to cover hair. Wrap head with a shower cap for 12 hours. Shampoo and comb out dead lice and eggs.
Psoriasis	1 part	1 part water	NA	Drink slowly morning and night.
Rashes	1 teaspoon	1 teaspoon water	NA	Dip cotton ball into vinegar and water and apply to affected area for 10 to 15 minutes. Rinse with water.
Ringworm	1 teaspoon	NA	NA	Apply to affected area directly up to six times a day.
Scarring	1 teaspoon	1 teaspoon water	NA	Dip cotton ball into vinegar and water and apply to scar tissue for 10 to 15 minutes. Rinse with water.
Shampoo buildup	1 tablespoon	1 cup	1 to 2 drops lemon essential oil	After shampooing, combine and rinse through hair.
Sore throat	1 teaspoon	½ cup water	Dash sea salt	Gargle mixture up to three times an hour, never swallowing.
Sunburn	1 cup	Bathtub of cool water	Aloe vera gel (optional)	Enjoy a cool bath up to 30 minutes, followed by vinegar directly applied to any affected areas.
Sun spots	1 part	NA	1 part macerated onion or onion juice	Apply with a cotton swab directly onto spots.
Thinning hair	2 tablespoons	2 tablespoons	Dash cayenne	Apply up to 10 minutes before shampooing.
Varicose veins	1 cup	NA	NA	Apply vinegar to the veins morning and night, using your hands in a cupping motion.
Warts	⅓ cup	Tub of water	NA	Soak affected area in warm mixture without rubbing. Apply vinegar-soaked bandage overnight.
Weak hair	⅓ cup	4 cups water	1 to 2 drops lavender essential oil	Rinse hair with mixture after shampooing, once every month.
Weight gain	2 teaspoons	1 cup water	NA	Drink at each meal.
Yellow teeth	3 teaspoons	1 cup	NA	Gargle 10 to 30 seconds. Rinse mouth well afterward.

FREQUENTLY ASKED QUESTIONS ABOUT APPLE CIDER VINEGAR

Can apple cider vinegar go bad? How do I properly store it?

Vinegars, by nature, are self-preserving. However, for best results, they should be kept in airtight, glass containers in a cool, dry place, away from direct sunlight. If your vinegar is raw and still contains live bacteria, keeping it in a cool, dark place, or even a refrigerator, will help halt further and unwanted fermentation. Pasteurized vinegars will keep indefinitely, but it's always a good idea to adhere to the "best by" date suggested by the manufacturer. Use your common sense . . . and your nose! If it smells rotten, throw it out.

What is the pH value of apple cider vinegar?

All liquids can be measured on a pH scale, which stands for potential hydrogen and measures the concentration of hydrogen ions in the liquid. A liquid is then determined to be either acidic (pH below 7.0) or alkaline (pH above 7.0). Distilled water is the exact neutral (7.0). Depending on the particular mixture or ferment, apple cider vinegar has been shown by different sources to have a pH anywhere from 2.0 to 7.0. Interestingly, when certain acids and bases combine, a by-product is often given off, which is why vinegar is combined with baking soda in some baking recipes to act as a rising agent.

Does it matter whether I purchase organic apple cider vinegar?

Yes! Each year the Environmental Working Group (EWG) publishes a guide to pesticides in produce. It's a list of the most pesticide-laden produce, known as the "Dirty Dozen" (see also Appendix B, page 200). Apples have made it to the top of that list for the fifth year in a row, meaning you should definitely spend the extra change to purchase apples that are certified organic. According to the EWG, apples are extra "dirty" because they contain chemicals applied both before and after harvest with the intent of longer preservation. These chemicals will be passed on from the apples to the vinegar. Look for organic apple cider vinegar, and use that in your remedies and recipes.

Is it possible to consume too much apple cider vinegar?

There are a few reports online from apple cider vinegar users who claim that their long-term use of a couple tablespoons a day resulted in a change in overall bone density, making it potentially dangerous to those with osteoporosis. There are also several reports of an over-consumption of apple cider vinegar, causing decreased potassium levels. To date, no official scientific studies have been published.

Is apple cider vinegar a probiotic?

Yes and no. An unpasteurized and unfiltered bottle of apple cider vinegar contains wispy filaments of probiotic bacteria, with the main clump (usually at the bottom) referred to as the mother. If you buy pasteurized vinegar, it will not have any probiotic benefits—any living nutrients will have been killed off in the high-heat pasteurization process.

The organic acids in apple cider vinegar encourage healthy gut flora, much like probiotics do, but the acids themselves are not probiotics. On the other hand, apple cider vinegar is made with an ingredient that encourages the growth of probiotics—apple pectin. One study found that pectin is what health professionals are beginning to refer to as a prebiotic. Prebiotics act as fertilizer for the probiotics already in your system. They encourage the growth of the good, probiotic bacteria.

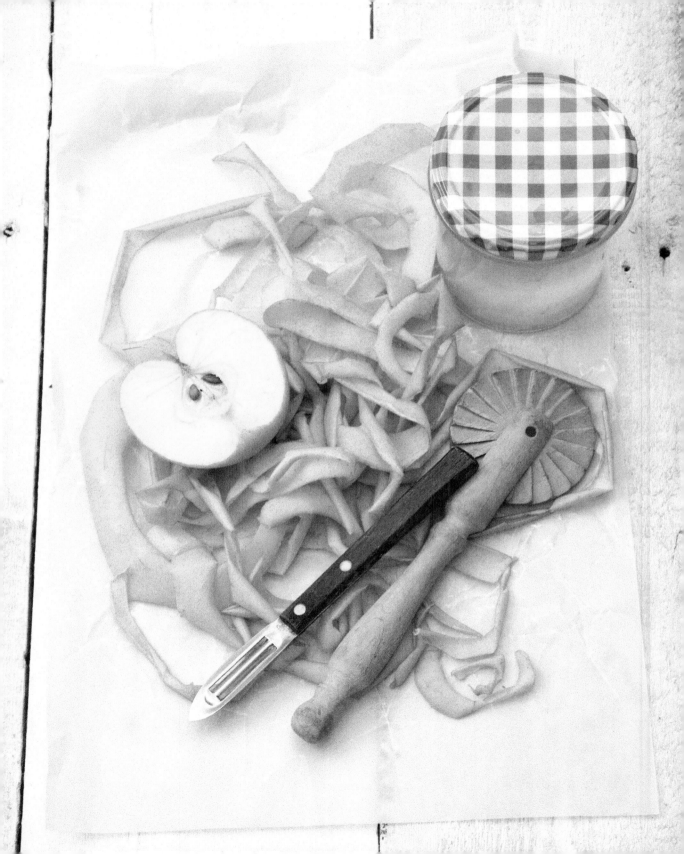

Chapter Three

HOMEMADE APPLE CIDER VINEGAR

WHILE IT IS POSSIBLE TO MAKE apple cider vinegar from a small sampling of raw vinegar and juice, the most healthful and nutrient-rich batch comes from the slow fermentation of actual fruit pieces. The simple apple contains all the elements necessary to produce an enzyme-rich, living serving of apple cider vinegar. We need only nudge it along on its transformation. The tannins from the skin give the finished product astringency, the organic acids provide sharp freshness, and the abundant bacteria in the air are patiently waiting to attack the alcohols before their conversion to vinegar. The process of making apple cider vinegar may be lengthy, but it's also quite easy. We hope you'll give it a go!

CORE INGREDIENTS

Vinegar amateurs may be pleasantly surprised to learn that apple cider vinegar does not require unusual ingredients. All you need for your first batch is water, apples, and sugar. Because the building blocks are minimal, make sure each is of high quality, pure, and organic, when possible.

Apples

With over 7,500 apple varieties grown in the world today, how do you choose the perfect apple as the base for vinegar? Some vinegar masters swear by their single-variety recipe, while others have been using their own special apple combinations for decades—often three or more types. Apples are as unique and varied as the people who eat them—some sweet, some sharp, some bitter. If you feel experimental, try a mixture of sweet and tangy to create a vinegar with more depth. Fuji and Gala apples are on the sweeter side of the spectrum, whereas McIntosh and Granny Smith are on the tart side.

Apples are the world's third most widely grown fruit (bananas are first, grapes second). They're a cooling food that promotes energy and inhibits fermentation in the stomach, which, as we've learned, encourages absorption of nutrients from our foods. They are a rich source of pectin, found predominantly in their skins. Pectin is a soluble plant fiber that supports a healthy digestive tract and acts as food for the good bacteria in your gut. Many of these nutritious benefits are transferred to your bottles of apple cider vinegar through the fermentation process.

Whichever unique apple variety you choose, it's vital that you choose organic apples and wash them well. As noted earlier, for five years running, apples have tested as the most pesticide-laden produce by the Environmental Working Group. Nonorganic apples also receive a waxy coating once harvested to protect them from spoiling; this wax consists of either carnauba or shellac made from insect secretions and food additive E904. And so, it's definitely worth the extra money to purchase apples that are certified organic.

Sugar or Honey

Pure cane sugar—or sucanat, an abbreviation for *sugar cane natural*—is recommended for the most efficient and healthy fermentation process. But honey is a perfectly acceptable alternative. Use organic raw honey, which contains live enzymes and bacteria that can assist in making your vinegar. Raw honey can be purchased at your local farmers' markets and at some health food stores. Honey has an indefinite shelf life, so don't be reluctant to stock up.

If you're worried about consuming too much sugar, keep in mind that the end result will be extremely low in sugar (consider how bitter vinegar tastes) because the small amount of sugar used is simply there to feed the hungry bacteria as they ferment the cider into vinegar. The main thing to avoid is the use of artificial sweeteners.

Water

As the base of your vinegar, it's important to start with filtered or distilled water. Many cities add chlorine or fluoride to their water, which can negatively affect the mother in your vinegar, as well as your vinegar's final taste. Avoid hard water, as well, by boiling it uncovered for at least 2 minutes and then letting it sit overnight—any mineral deposits will separate and sink to the bottom. Then gently ladle the water from the top so as not to disrupt any unwanted sediment on the bottom of the pot.

ESSENTIAL EQUIPMENT

You don't need to invest in the most expensive fermentation equipment right from the start—use what you have at home until you get into a regular fermenting groove. Our ancestors made all types of vinegars without any of the new-fangled appliances on the market today, so take a lesson from those who have gone before us and start small. Here are the basics for getting started.

Brewing Container

Choose a clean glass container in which to begin your ferment, such as a quart mason jar or a gallon glass cookie jar or candy jar, depending on how big your first brew is. The jar doesn't need a lid, but needs to have a wide enough mouth to accommodate rough cuts of apple. A wider jar also encourages more oxygen exchange, since the surface area of the liquid will be wider. Glass is important when working with any acidic concoction, such as vinegar, so no chemicals or toxins can leach into your ferment from its walls. Any reactive metal (aluminum, copper, iron, or steel) touching the vinegar will not only make the liquid unfit to drink; it could also make it taste "off." You can also use nonleaded ceramic, such as the insert to most slow cooker appliances, although that may be too large for your first at-home batch.

Clean Cotton Cloth

This cotton cloth will be the single barrier between your prized vinegar and the hungry fruit flies and ants that will surely come looking for a taste. If you use cheesecloth, you may need to double or triple the layers. The holes in cheesecloth are more porous than common cotton cloths like a kitchen towel, T-shirt, or pillowcase. Whatever you use, make sure it's clean and well secured with a rubber band over the rim of the container.

Strainer

You'll need a strainer for when you strain the ripened vinegar from the mother and remaining apple particles. Our first recommendation is a doubled piece of cheesecloth, but you can also use a fine-mesh sieve. Although sometimes made from metal, the time it interacts with the vinegar is negligible.

Storage Containers

Store your vinegar in a glass container with a narrower neck than the jars you made it in. This helps halt fermentation by restricting the amount of oxygen touching the surface of the vinegar. Flip-top glass bottles are a favorite among fermentation experts because they can withstand pressure, they're reusable, and they don't require any special type of capping mechanism. If you choose to store your finished vinegar in a container with a screw-on lid, such as a mason jar, get nonreactive lids. These can be purchased online, or at a brewer's supply store, or wherever canning equipment is sold.

EVALUATING AND BOTTLING YOUR VINEGAR

The time has finally come to assess your vinegar creation! When evaluating your homemade vinegar, it really comes down to tasting and seeing. Good apple cider vinegar should never taste or smell putrid. If it does, trust your instincts and throw it out. Refer to our troubleshooting section (see page 36) for common problems that may have occurred in your batch. Don't give up! Make some adjustments in your approach and try again.

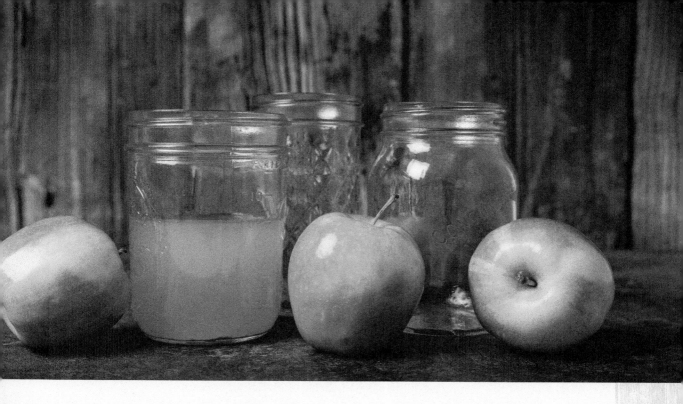

Fermenting Environment

While the fermentation of apple cider vinegar can feel like a finicky project with lots of specific requirements, most of these tasks can easily be carried out in the average home kitchen.

STERILIZATION: To produce the best apple cider vinegar, it's crucial that you begin with a sterilized environment and equipment. This goes for the starting containers, the cloth cover, and final bottling equipment.

TEMPERATURE: The temperature for the waiting period of your fermentation process should be as constant as possible, hovering between 60°F and 80°F. If the temperature in your home rises higher than this during the day, or drops sharply at night, consider investing in a special heated mat or container jacket made specifically for fermentation.

SUNLIGHT: Keeping your ferment out of direct sunlight is fundamental to the well-being of the mother and other wisps of bacteria that give birth to your vinegar. Direct sunlight can cause excessive heat and should be avoided.

FINISHED FERMENTS: To put a grand halt to further fermentation (which could lead to a vinegar that's too strong for consumption), keep raw, homemade apple cider vinegar in the refrigerator. If sealed properly, you can also store finished ferments in a cool room in your house, preferably between 38°F and 50°F. Freezing is not recommended for extended storage, since this will kill any benefits you could receive from the vinegar's probiotic material or raw enzymes.

If your finished product tastes "just okay," don't lose heart. Most vinegar will benefit from a little aging, so don't be afraid to make an extra-large batch your first time and store some away for several months in order to taste test the difference. The longer vinegar is left to age, the mellower and more mature its flavor profile becomes.

TROUBLESHOOTING GUIDE

Trust your gut when it comes to the fermentation process. You may need to tweak a thing or two, but over time and with a little experience, you'll work out the kinks. Taking notes is a great practice to develop in the kitchen; jot down what works and doesn't work for you. In the meantime, here are some obstacles you may face and tips to overcome them in the quest for homemade vinegar:

Fruit Flies

Due to the sweet nature of the ingredients, your brewing batch of apple cider vinegar may attract fruit flies and other sweet-toothed insects. You can fight back using a double piece of cheesecloth fabric, or securing the cloth with a tighter rubber band. Another option is to keep your fermenting jar(s) in a warm, bug-free room away from windows or access points for fruit flies to enter. You can also place a small dish of sweet vinegar in another area of the room or house to attract the little bugs elsewhere. Remember, all it takes is one rebel fruit fly entering the jar to produce an entire family in your vinegar! Once infested, you'll need to throw out that batch and begin again.

Mold

Don't mistake your vinegar's growing mother for mold. Be sure to do some image searching online to compare potential mold notes with other vinegar makers before you toss your batch. Mold in an apple cider vinegar ferment is rarer than you may think, thanks to the naturally acidic environment of your creation, but it can occur when temperatures are too low or your mother isn't strong enough and dies off.

"Off" Flavors

If your end result doesn't taste quite right, it could be due to a number of causes. What's your water like? If your city adds chlorine or fluoride to its water, this can add a funky taste to your vinegar, while also killing the necessary bacteria for fermentation. Hard water that leaves lines in your sinks, showers, and toilets will also make a less appealing vinegar. To distill your own tap water, simply bring it to a boil, uncovered, for at least 2 minutes, and then let it sit overnight. The chlorine will vaporize, and any mineral deposits will separate and sink to the bottom. Gently ladle the water from the top so as not to disrupt any unwanted sediment on the bottom of the pot.

In addition, if you're on a fermentation roll and have other ferments (kombucha, pickles, sourdough bread) fermenting nearby on your countertop, the airborne bacteria may intermingle where you don't want them to, making for a foul-tasting apple cider vinegar batch.

HOMEMADE APPLE CIDER VINEGAR

MAKES: 1 QUART • PREP TIME: 10 MINUTES • FERMENTATION TIME: 4 TO 5 WEEKS

Making your own apple cider vinegar is both practical and educational. You'll witness firsthand how the raw ingredients change when given enough time and a little help from the magic of fermentation. If you want the freshest, purest and most potent vinegar available to you, choose your ingredients carefully and use the recipe below to craft your own amber-colored concoction for use in cooking, healing, or body care.

3¾ cups water

¼ cup raw honey

2 medium, ripe apples, cut into chunks, or the scraps (flesh, peel, cores) from 4 apples

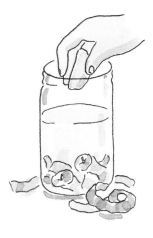

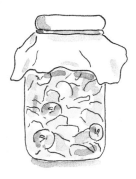

1. In a large glass jar, stir together the water and honey until completely dissolved. Add the apples.

2. Securely cover the jar with a clean cotton towel or cloth, and place it in a warm location.

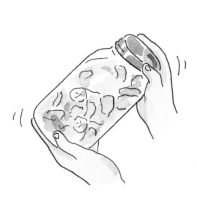

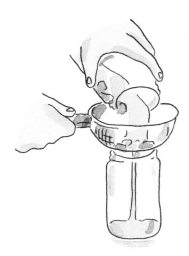

3. Shake the jar once every day to agitate the ingredients.

4. After about 1 week, the alcohol fermentation stage will end and the apple pieces will fall to the bottom of the jar. Strain the apple pieces from the liquid, which is now hard cider, and return the cider to a sanitized jar.

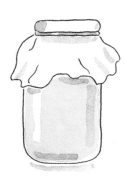

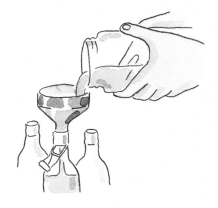

5. Cover the jar with a clean cotton towel or cloth again, and place it in a warm location. After 3 to 4 weeks, the vinegar should be ready. Do a smell test and a taste test to determine its status. If it needs more time, wait another week and test it again.

6. When ready, bottle the vinegar in a sanitized glass bottle with an airtight nonreactive lid. Store in a cool, dark place.

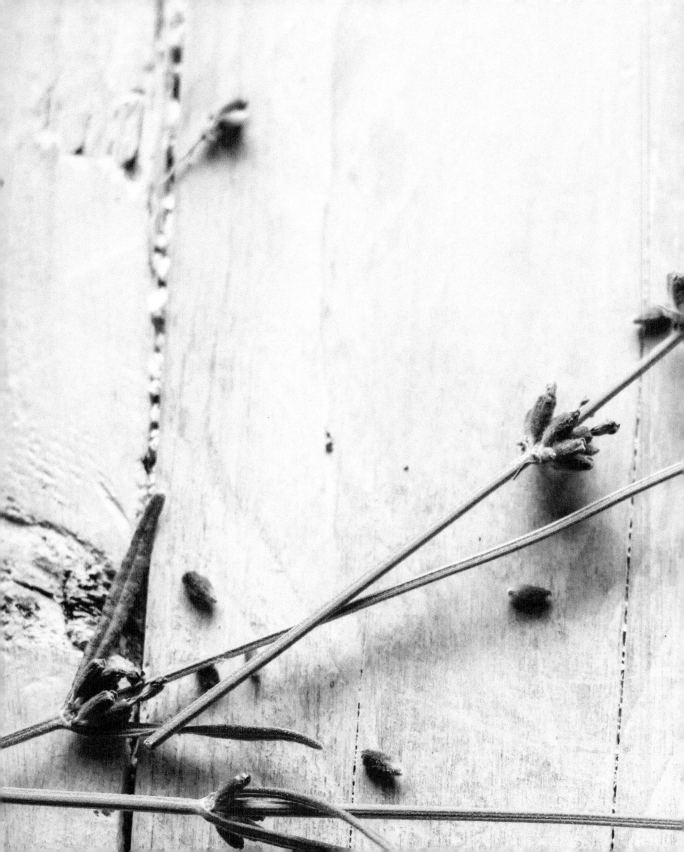

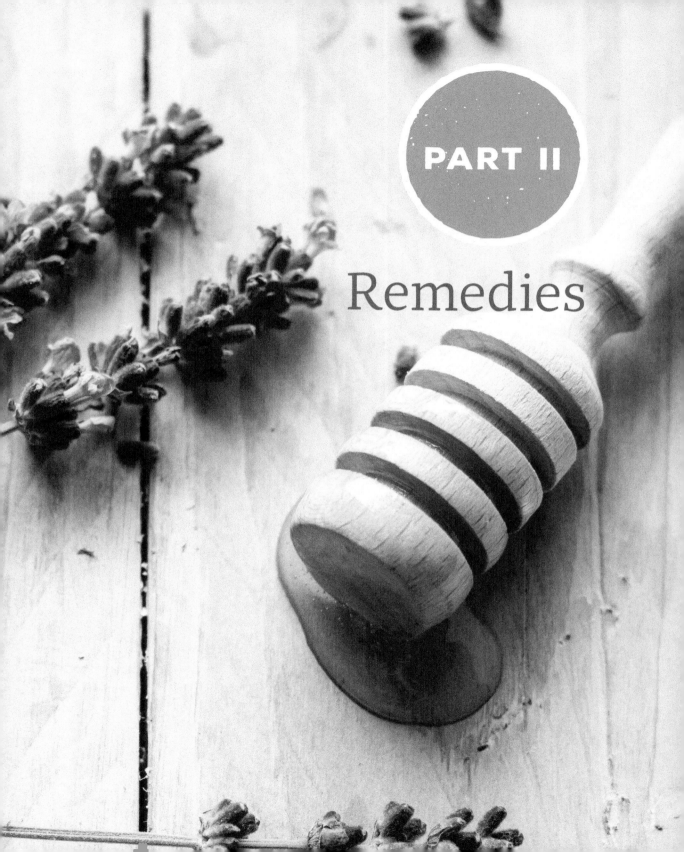

PART II

Remedies

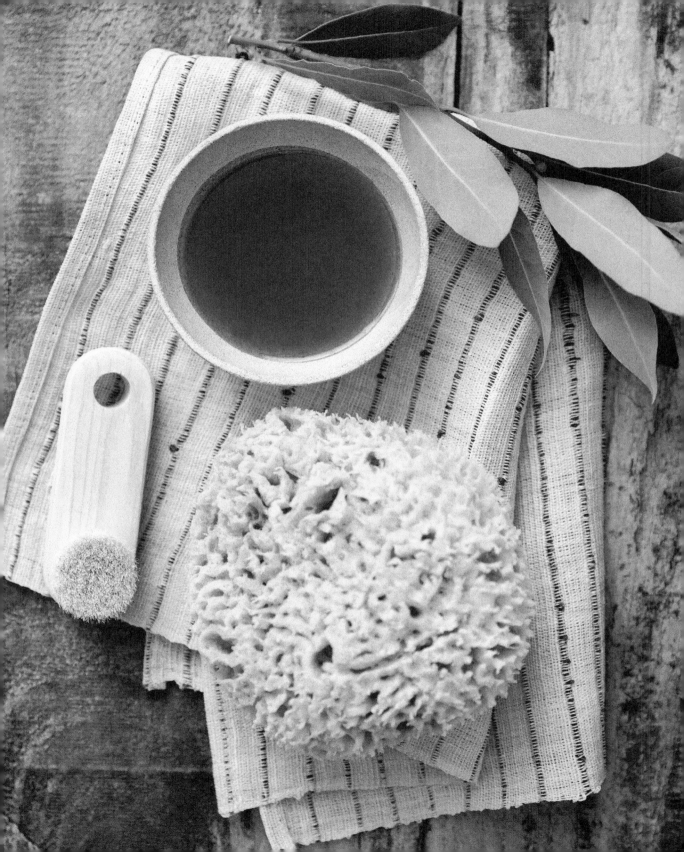

Chapter Four

BODY & HAIR CARE

44 Acne
Basic Apple Cider Vinegar Facial Toner
Pumpkin Pie Enzyme Mask
Activated Charcoal and Clay Facial Pack

46 Dandruff
Nettle and Tea Tree Rinse
Exfoliating Lemon-Sugar Scalp Scrub

48 Dry Skin
Castor Oil and Witch Hazel Makeup Remover
Rosewater and Sea Salt Body Spray
Mango Skin Slougher

50 Foot Care
Lime and Mint Salt Scrub
Cracked Heel Salve with Rice
Antifungal Tea Tree Nail Soak

52 Hand Care
Pre-Mani Nail Soak
Lemon-Lavender Hand Spray

54 Hyperpigmentation
Aloe Vera-Turmeric Gel Facial
Applesauce and Papaya Purée Peel
Lip-Lightening Paste

56 Sunburn
Parched Skin Peppermint Spray
Lavender-Oatmeal Soak

58 Varicose Veins
Citrus Cypress Spray
Magnesium Massage Oil
Rosemary–Epsom Salts Soak

60 Dry Hair
Chamomile Conditioning Rinse
Lavender-Coconut Hair Mask
Hair-Shining Tea and Sea Spray

62 Oily Hair
Lavender Scalp Toner
Cucumber-Lemon Cleanser

ACNE

Whether the cause is diet, hormones, or genetics, acne affects the majority of the population at one time or another. And age, sadly, doesn't always seem to be a cure for it! Thankfully, natural remedies like apple cider vinegar boast mighty healing benefits without the side effects that many medications bring. The acetic acid in apple cider vinegar works to restore our skin's natural acid mantle, while dissolving dead skin cells and killing acne-causing bacteria.

BASIC APPLE CIDER VINEGAR FACIAL TONER

YIELD: 8 OUNCES
STORAGE: SEALED GLASS BOTTLE
PREP TIME: 1 MINUTE

Choosing raw, organic apple cider vinegar with all of its enzymes pure and intact is crucial to the effectiveness of this toner as well as the other remedies. Our skin is naturally acidic, and many mainstream facial products actually strip our skin of its ideal pH.

2 tablespoons apple cider vinegar
1 cup filtered water, plus more as needed

1. Add the vinegar to a glass bottle and top it off with filtered water. Cover and shake well.
2. To use, wet an organic cotton ball with the mixture and swipe gently over the face or problem areas before applying any moisturizer.

PUMPKIN PIE ENZYME MASK

YIELD: 1 TREATMENT
STORAGE: NOT RECOMMENDED
PREP TIME: 4 MINUTES
TREATMENT TIME: 10 MINUTES

Pumpkin is packed with the skin-smoothing antioxidant vitamins A and C, as well as powerful fruit enzymes and alpha-hydroxy acids to brighten skin naturally.

¼ cup cooked pumpkin, or canned pumpkin

1 tablespoon apple cider vinegar

1 teaspoon vitamin E oil

5 drops orange essential oil

½ teaspoon ground cinnamon

½ teaspoon ground ginger

½ teaspoon ground nutmeg

1. In a small nonreactive bowl, stir together the pumpkin, cider vinegar, vitamin E oil, orange essential oil, cinnamon, ginger, and nutmeg.

2. Spread a smooth layer on your face and allow it to dry for about 10 minutes.

3. Wash off with cool water.

4. Use 2 or 3 times a week, or as needed.

ACTIVATED CHARCOAL AND CLAY FACIAL PACK

YIELD: 1 TREATMENT
STORAGE: NOT RECOMMENDED
PREP TIME: 1 MINUTE
TREATMENT TIME: 15 MINUTES

The activated charcoal and clay in this recipe work together beautifully to draw out unwanted toxins from the skin. Activated charcoal is carbon that has been heated until it expands and becomes extremely porous, giving it the ability to trap any harmful waste your skin needs to get rid of.

1 tablespoon bentonite clay

1 tablespoon activated charcoal

Apple cider vinegar, for making a paste

1. In a small nonreactive container, mix together the bentonite clay, activated charcoal, and just enough apple cider vinegar to form a paste.

2. Apply a thick layer to your face, avoiding the eye area.

3. Leave on for about 15 minutes, or until dried.

4. Rinse off with warm water and pat the skin dry.

DANDRUFF

People with dandruff have an unusually rapid skin cell turnover rate, resulting in the common flakes of dead skin littering the scalp, hair, neck, and shoulder area. Causes range from dry skin and psoriasis to an overproduction of sebum, or skin oil. Try the following remedies on your quest to slough off dead skin and wear those dark shirts proudly again.

NETTLE AND TEA TREE RINSE

YIELD: 1 TREATMENT
STORAGE: LARGE SQUEEZE BOTTLE
PREP TIME: 30 MINUTES
TREATMENT TIME: 5 MINUTES

Nettle is a nutrient-dense plant, brimming with calcium, vitamins A and K, and protein, as well as many trace minerals like selenium, sulfur, and zinc. Tea tree oil is a naturally antiseptic essential oil bursting with both antifungal and antiviral benefits used historically to heal skin and scalp issues.

3 cups water
¼ cup dried nettle
1 tablespoon apple cider vinegar
2 or 3 drops tea tree essential oil

1. In a medium saucepan, bring the water to a boil. Remove from the heat.

2. Add the nettle and stir to combine. Steep for at least 15 minutes.

3. Using a fine-mesh sieve, strain out the nettle and discard. Cool the liquid.

4. Pour the cooled liquid into a large squeeze bottle. Add the cider vinegar and tea tree oil. Cover and shake to combine.

5. In the shower, pour the mixture onto all sections of your scalp, massaging as you go. Once all is applied, let sit for 5 minutes.

6. Rinse well.

EXFOLIATING LEMON-SUGAR SCALP SCRUB

YIELD: 1 TREATMENT
STORAGE: NOT RECOMMENDED
PREP TIME: 2 MINUTES
TREATMENT TIME: 5 MINUTES

The lemon in this remedy provides citric acid that naturally tones the scalp and rids it of unwanted dead skin cells.

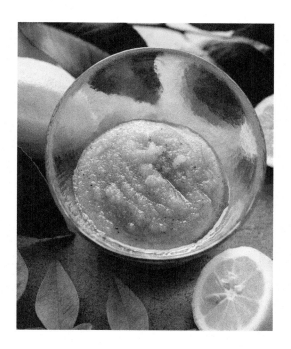

2 tablespoons brown sugar or sucanat

2 tablespoons argan oil or coconut oil

2 tablespoons apple cider vinegar

2 tablespoons freshly squeezed lemon juice, or 2 to 5 drops lemon essential oil

1. In a small nonreactive bowl, combine the brown sugar, argan oil, cider vinegar, and lemon juice.

2. With your fingers, scoop out small amounts and work the scrub into your scalp with small circular motions for 5 minutes. Rinse thoroughly. Shampoo as usual.

DRY SKIN

Itchy, dry skin be gone! Winter typically brings on cracked and chapped skin, but these moisturizing recipes will heal dry skin in winter or any season, while working to further protect your epidermis from the harsh elements.

CASTOR OIL AND WITCH HAZEL MAKEUP REMOVER

YIELD: 4 OUNCES
STORAGE: SEALED GLASS BOTTLE
PREP TIME: 2 MINUTES

Witch hazel is a flowering shrub. The liquid witch hazel you buy at the drugstore is made from the leaves, bark, and twigs of the shrub and water. It is widely considered a natural skin astringent. In this recipe, it helps rid the top skin layers of unwanted dirt and makeup.

2 tablespoons witch hazel

2 tablespoons apple cider vinegar

2 tablespoons castor oil

2 tablespoons filtered water

2 to 5 drops carrot seed essential oil

1. In a glass bottle, combine the witch hazel, cider vinegar, castor oil, water, and carrot seed essential oil. Cover and shake to combine.

2. Shake before each use. Using a round cotton pad or cotton ball soaked with the solution, swipe across the face to remove dirt and makeup.

ROSEWATER AND SEA SALT BODY SPRAY

YIELD: 8 OUNCES
STORAGE: GLASS SPRAY BOTTLE
PREP TIME: 10 MINUTES

Essence of rose is subtle and sweet, and it possesses powerful soothing properties that moisturize and reduce redness in the skin. Trace mineral drops are an all-natural mineral supplement in concentrate form that can be used diluted on the skin to nourish from the outside in.

Scant 1 cup very hot water, or pure rosewater

1 rose tea bag, if not using pure rosewater

1 tablespoon sea salt

1 tablespoon aloe vera gel

1 tablespoon apple cider vinegar

2 or 3 drops trace minerals

2 or 3 drops lavender essential oil

1. In a small nonreactive bowl, combine the hot water and tea bag. Steep for 5 minutes. Remove the tea bag and discard.

2. Add the sea salt and stir until dissolved. Cool.

3. In a reusable spray bottle, combine the aloe vera gel, cider vinegar, trace minerals, and lavender essential oil. Fill the bottle with the cooled rose tea and sea salt liquid. Cover and shake well.

4. Keep refrigerated. Spray on dry skin, as needed.

MANGO SKIN SLOUGHER

YIELD: 1 TREATMENT
STORAGE: NOT RECOMMENDED
PREP TIME: 5 MINUTES
TREATMENT TIME: 10 MINUTES

Mangos contain mangiferin, a natural bioactive compound full of antioxidant activity that protects against skin damage. Mangos also contain vitamin A, which renews the skin without the irritating side effects that some commercial Retin-A creams bring. Honey is a natural humectant that works to retain moisture.

1 mango, chopped

2 tablespoons oats

1 tablespoon apple cider vinegar

1 teaspoon raw honey

1. In a food processor or blender, purée the mango.

2. Add the oats, cider vinegar, and honey. Gently pulse for 3 seconds to combine. The mixture should retain some of the bulk and roughness of the oats.

3. In the shower, use the full amount on your entire body: first as a scrub for 3 minutes, and then as a mask, leaving it on for 5 to 7 minutes.

4. Rinse with warm water.

FOOT CARE

Feet—our humble warriors—take the brunt of our work and weight throughout the day. Treat your toes (and heels) to a little TLC with these scrubs, salves, and soaks that not only smell scrumptious, but get rid of fungus and other foot ailments as well.

LIME AND MINT SALT SCRUB

YIELD: ABOUT 8 TREATMENTS
STORAGE: SEALED GLASS JAR
PREP TIME: 5 MINUTES

Moisturize your feet while sloughing off dead skin and calluses with the help of some thick-grained Epsom salts. The minerals in the salts work to soften tough skin while relaxing the muscles. A carrier oil is any base oil derived from the fatty portion of a plant that is used to dilute and carry essential oils to the skin.

¼ cup olive oil, avocado oil, or other carrier oil

5 drops lime essential oil

2 drops peppermint essential oil

2 drops wintergreen essential oil

2 tablespoons apple cider vinegar

¾ cup Epsom salts

1. Add the olive oil to a medium nonreactive bowl.

2. Whisk in the lime essential oil, peppermint essential oil, wintergreen essential oil, and cider vinegar.

3. Slowly whisk in the Epsom salts until well combined.

4. In the bath or shower, apply about 1 tablespoon per foot, rubbing for about 5 minutes with a pumice stone or washcloth.

   Note: Use with caution, as ingredients may cause tub or shower floor to become slippery.

CRACKED HEEL SALVE WITH RICE

YIELD: ABOUT 8 TREATMENTS
STORAGE: SEALED GLASS JAR
PREP TIME: 5 MINUTES
TREATMENT TIME: 20 MINUTES

This salve is fun to whip up. It uses rice, one of our most common dinner ingredients, as an exfoliant! Geranium oil is medicinally known to revitalize old body tissues, so it should be a welcome relief to your overworked heels.

¾ cup dry rice
2 tablespoons raw honey
1 tablespoon apple cider vinegar
5 drops geranium essential oil
Coconut oil, for treating (optional)

1. In the blender, pulse the rice until it reaches a semicoarse flour consistency.

2. Add the honey, cider vinegar, and geranium essential oil. Process into a paste.

3. Soak your feet in a tub of warm water for at least 15 minutes.

4. Apply the paste generously, about 1 tablespoon per foot, to any dry or cracked areas, rubbing gently with a pumice stone, washcloth, or your hand for about 5 minutes.

5. Rinse with warm water.

6. Repeat every few days until skin of your heels fully heals, applying a layer of coconut oil after each treatment (if using).

ANTIFUNGAL TEA TREE NAIL SOAK

YIELD: 1 TREATMENT
STORAGE: NOT RECOMMENDED
PREP TIME: 2 MINUTES
TREATMENT TIME: 20 TO 30 MINUTES

The vinegar and tea tree oil in this remedy work synergistically to kill nail fungus, while the baking soda will stand guard, ensuring no fungus grows or spreads in the future.

Warm water, for soaking
1 cup apple cider vinegar
5 drops tea tree essential oil
5 tablespoons baking soda

1. Fill a foot-soaking tub with warm water and put it someplace where you can sit comfortably.

2. Add the cider vinegar and tea tree essential oil and stir to combine.

3. Soak your feet in the warm mixture for 10 to 15 minutes.

4. Dry your feet well, rubbing to remove any dead skin or fungus that has sloughed off.

5. Add the baking soda to the water and stir to combine.

6. Soak your feet for another 10 to 15 minutes to prevent the spread of fungus. Dry your feet thoroughly.

HAND CARE

We use our hands almost every minute of every day. So, next time you need a little self-love, give your hands some extra care. Hand care doesn't have to end in pretty, painted nails—simply exposing your nails and cuticles to a few key ingredients can make a big difference in how they look and feel.

PRE-MANI NAIL SOAK

YIELD: 1 TREATMENT
STORAGE: NOT RECOMMENDED
PREP TIME: 2 MINUTES
TREATMENT TIME: 10 MINUTES

Carrot seed oil is one of the top essential oils that promotes shine, smoothness, and strength in nails. Its benefits far outweigh its earthy scent, but if you dislike the smell, add a few drops of lavender essential oil to the mix.

Warm water, for soaking

1 tablespoon olive oil

2 to 3 drops carrot seed essential oil

1 tablespoon apple cider vinegar, plus more as needed

1. Add enough warm water to a medium glass bowl so all fingernails fit beneath the liquid.

2. Stir in the olive oil, carrot seed essential oil, and cider vinegar.

3. Immerse your fingers in the bowl. Soak for up to 10 minutes.

4. Remove your hands and dry well.

5. If painting your nails, first dip a cotton ball in cider vinegar and swipe across your nails to remove any oil that might disrupt the adhesion of the polish.

LEMON-LAVENDER HAND SPRAY

YIELD: 4 OUNCES
STORAGE: GLASS SPRAY BOTTLE
PREP TIME: 5 MINUTES

Frequent nail massages with olive oil and lemon essential oil promote nail growth and make brittle nails a thing of the past. If you have any nail fungus on your hands, this spray will get rid of that too.

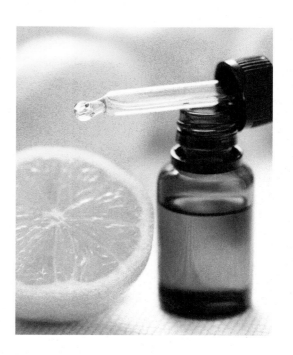

2 tablespoons olive oil

1 tablespoon jojoba oil

1 tablespoon apple cider vinegar

1 teaspoon vitamin E oil

2 to 5 drops lavender essential oil

2 to 5 drops lemon essential oil

1. In a glass spray bottle, combine the olive oil, jojoba oil, cider vinegar, vitamin E oil, lavender essential oil, and lemon essential oil. Cover and shake well.

2. Before bed, spray the mixture on your hands, and rub it in thoroughly for 5 minutes. Pay special attention to the nail beds and cuticles, because the massage increases circulation and promotes nail health and growth.

3. Use throughout the day as a natural hand disinfectant. The essential oils and vinegar work together to kill any bacteria and fungus present.

HYPERPIGMENTATION

There are three main types of hyperpigmentation, or dark skin spots, each associated with a different cause. Age spots stem from sun exposure; melasma is brought on by pregnancy, or sometimes birth control hormones; and, post-inflammatory marks are left behind after acne or a bug bite heals.

ALOE VERA-TURMERIC GEL FACIAL

YIELD: 1 TREATMENT
STORAGE: NOT RECOMMENDED
PREP TIME: 4 MINUTES
TREATMENT TIME: 10 MINUTES

While each ingredient in this gel facial has unique skin-lightening abilities, the aloe vera gel base, in particular, is a gentle yet effective lightener. Its mucilaginous polysaccharides remove dead skin and promote skin cell regeneration.

¼ cup aloe vera gel

1 tablespoon apple cider vinegar

1 teaspoon vitamin E oil

½ teaspoon ground turmeric

2 drops lemon essential oil

2 drops orange essential oil

1. In a small nonreactive bowl, combine the aloe vera gel, cider vinegar, vitamin E oil, turmeric, lemon essential oil, and orange essential oil. Mix well.

2. Spread a smooth layer on your face and allow it to dry for 10 minutes.

3. Wash off with cool water.

4. Use 2 to 3 times a week, or as needed.

APPLESAUCE AND PAPAYA PURÉE PEEL

YIELD: 1 TREATMENT
STORAGE: NOT RECOMMENDED
PREP TIME: 5 MINUTES
TREATMENT TIME: 15 MINUTES

Apples contain a good amount of malic acid, which helps even out facial skin complexion and get rid of age spots. Papayas contain papain, an enzyme that will immediately go to work to renew the top layer of your skin— you may even feel a slight refreshing tingle.

---

1 tablespoon applesauce, preferably organic
1 tablespoon raw papaya
1 teaspoon apple cider vinegar

1. In a small nonreactive bowl, mash together the applesauce, papaya, and cider vinegar. Stir until well combined.
2. With clean hands or a face brush, apply the mixture to your face, avoiding the eye area. Let sit for 10 to 15 minutes.
3. Remove with a soft cloth and cool water.

LIP-LIGHTENING PASTE

YIELD: ABOUT 1 OUNCE
STORAGE: REFRIGERATE IN A SEALED GLASS CONTAINER
PREP TIME: 5 MINUTES
TREATMENT TIME: 10 MINUTES

Raspberries not only contain vital vitamins and minerals for your internal organs, but they also work wonders on your skin. Combined with almond oil, they will begin to work their magic immediately. Don't leave this paste on too long or it will temporarily dye your lips pink—unless you like that look, of course!

---

2 or 3 fresh raspberries, washed
1 teaspoon apple cider vinegar
1 teaspoon sweet almond oil
Few drops raw honey (optional)

1. In a small nonreactive bowl, mash the raspberries.
2. Stir in the cider vinegar, sweet almond oil, and honey (if using). Mix until a paste forms.
3. Massage the paste onto your lips and let sit for up to 10 minutes.
4. Rinse off and apply a natural moisturizer.

SUNBURN

Get caught in the sun too long? Forgot the proper SPF? It happens to the best of us. Avoid the awful repercussions associated with sunburned skin with these soothing, calming, and moisture-inducing remedies. Use after a long day outside to calm sun-kissed skin or to soothe a fully developed sunburn. Your red-hot skin will be encouraged to heal quickly and painlessly.

PARCHED SKIN PEPPERMINT SPRAY

YIELD: 8 OUNCES
STORAGE: GLASS SPRAY BOTTLE
PREP TIME: 15 MINUTES

An antioxidant powerhouse, green tea reduces post-sun skin inflammation thanks to the phytochemical and anticarcinogen epigallocatechin-3-gallate *(ECGC).*

---

2 cups water
1 chamomile tea bag
1 green tea bag
2 tablespoons aloe vera gel
1 tablespoon avocado oil or sweet almond oil
1 tablespoon apple cider vinegar
1 teaspoon sea salt
15 drops peppermint essential oil
15 drops lavender essential oil

1. In a small nonreactive saucepan set over high heat, bring the water to a boil. Remove from the heat. Add the chamomile tea bag and green tea bag and steep for 10 minutes. Discard the tea bags. Cool completely.

2. In a spray bottle, combine the aloe vera gel, avocado oil, cider vinegar, sea salt, peppermint essential oil, and lavender essential oil.

3. Top the spray bottle off with the cooled tea. Cover and shake to combine. (Refrigerate any leftover tea to drink or make more skin spray within 2 weeks.)

4. Refrigerate for up to 1 month.

5. Shake before each use.

LAVENDER-OATMEAL SOAK

YIELD: 1 TREATMENT
STORAGE: NOT RECOMMENDED
PREP TIME: 5 MINUTES
TREATMENT TIME: 30 MINUTES

Oats are the perfect chemical-free way to treat sunburn. They have anti-inflammatory properties and are full of antioxidants that soothe all kinds of skin irritations.

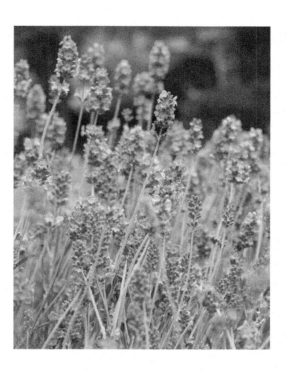

2 cups ground oats

½ cup baking soda

1 cup apple cider vinegar

2 tablespoons raw honey

5 drops lavender essential oil

1. Fill a bathtub with tepid water—as cool as you can tolerate.

2. In a piece of muslin cloth or a clean cotton sock, combine the oats and baking soda. Tie shut.

3. Toss the oat bundle into the filled tub. Add the cider vinegar, honey, and lavender essential oil and stir to distribute.

4. Soak in the tub and relax for up to 30 minutes.

5. Rinse off completely, pat dry, and moisturize.

VARICOSE VEINS

Varicose (or spider) veins are caused by damaged blood vessels resulting in dark places of stagnant blood under the skin. This poor circulation is often associated with leg pain and aches. In addition to using these home remedies, elevate your legs throughout the day as often as possible and sleep with your legs slightly propped up on a pillow.

CITRUS CYPRESS SPRAY

YIELD: ABOUT 4 OUNCES
STORAGE: GLASS SPRAY BOTTLE
PREP TIME: 5 MINUTES
TREATMENT TIME: 5 MINUTES

Cypress oil, taken from its evergreen tree namesake, has a fresh, woodsy scent. It has been used medicinally for centuries to heal a multitude of ailments. This remedy works effectively to regulate blood flow and relax muscles.

⅓ cup witch hazel
2 tablespoons apple cider vinegar
10 drops cypress essential oil
10 drops lemon essential oil
Water, for mixing

1. In a glass spray bottle, combine the witch hazel, cider vinegar, cypress essential oil, and lemon essential oil.

2. Top off the bottle with water. Cover and shake well.

3. Spritz on legs and other problem areas morning and night, massaging lightly for 5 minutes to encourage circulation.

MAGNESIUM MASSAGE OIL

YIELD: ABOUT 8 OUNCES
STORAGE: GLASS SPRAY BOTTLE
PREP TIME: 10 MINUTES
TREATMENT TIME: 5 MINUTES

Magnesium is best absorbed through the skin. Tingling is normal at first. Helichrysum oil, though expensive, is a potent antioxidant-rich oil known for reducing blood clots and healing circulatory disorders.

¼ cup water

¼ cup magnesium chloride flakes

2 tablespoons apple cider vinegar

2 tablespoons jojoba oil

2 tablespoons vitamin E oil

10 drops lavender essential oil

10 drops helichrysum essential oil (optional)

1. In a small nonreactive saucepan set over high heat, bring the water to a boil.

2. Add the magnesium flakes and stir until dissolved. Remove from the heat and cool.

3. In a glass spray bottle, combine the cider vinegar, jojoba oil, vitamin E oil, lavender essential oil, and helichrysum essential oil (if using).

4. Top off the bottle with the magnesium water. Cover and shake well.

5. Shake well before each use. Apply to the legs (and other problem areas) by spraying on a thin layer. Massage into your legs for 5 minutes, moving upward toward the heart.

ROSEMARY–EPSOM SALTS SOAK

YIELD: 1 TREATMENT
STORAGE: NOT RECOMMENDED
PREP TIME: 5 MINUTES
TREATMENT TIME: 15 MINUTES

Excessive exposure to heat or lengthy hot baths can lead to vein swelling. So keep the soaking time under 15 minutes or simply settle for a warm water temperature. The herbs and salts in this remedy work together to relax blood vessels and thereby reduce spider veins.

½ cup dried calendula flowers

½ cup Epsom salts

½ cup apple cider vinegar

10 drops rosemary essential oil

1. While drawing a tub of warm water, place the dried calendula flowers in a piece of cheesecloth or small muslin cloth bag, and tie to secure.

2. Toss the calendula flower bundle into the full tub. Add the Epsom salts, cider vinegar, and rosemary essential oil and swirl to distribute.

3. Soak up to 15 minutes in the tub, with your legs elevated above your heart.

4. To further increase circulation, rinse your legs with very cold water.

DRY HAIR

If you're looking to trade in your brittle, breaking locks for shiny, smooth tresses, make apple cider vinegar a permanent fixture on your shower rack. The acidity is pH balancing to your hair, closing up the cuticle's scales as it drips down each hair follicle.

CHAMOMILE CONDITIONING RINSE

YIELD: 1 TREATMENT
STORAGE: LARGE SQUEEZE BOTTLE
PREP TIME: 20 MINUTES, PLUS COOLING
TREATMENT TIME: 5 MINUTES

The chamomile in this floral-smelling hair rinse is a natural emollient, increasing hydration to hair follicles while making hair more pliable overall.

3 cups water

2 chamomile tea bags

3 tablespoons apple cider vinegar

2 to 3 drops lavender essential oil

1. In a medium nonreactive saucepan set over high heat, bring the water to a boil. Remove from the heat.

2. Add the tea bags and steep for at least 15 minutes. Discard the tea bags. Cool.

3. Pour the liquid into a large squeeze bottle. Add the cider vinegar and lavender essential oil. Cover and shake to combine.

4. In the shower, pour onto your hair and massage into your scalp. Let sit for 5 minutes. Rinse well.

LAVENDER-COCONUT HAIR MASK

YIELD: 1 TREATMENT
STORAGE: NOT RECOMMENDED
PREP TIME: 5 MINUTES
TREATMENT TIME: 10 MINUTES

The coconut oil in this mask seals in hair moisture, while the lavender oil has nutrients that penetrate deep into the follicles while removing buildup from other hair products.

3 tablespoons coconut oil
3 tablespoons raw honey
2 tablespoons apple cider vinegar
5 drops lavender essential oil

1. In a small nonreactive saucepan set over low heat, stir together the coconut oil and honey for 1 to 2 minutes, or until just melted. Remove from the heat.

2. Stir in the cider vinegar and lavender essential oil. Ingredients will begin to separate as they cool, so work quickly.

3. Work the mixture into your hair as you would a shampoo.

4. Let sit for 10 minutes before rinsing thoroughly.

HAIR-SHINING TEA AND SEA SPRAY

YIELD: ABOUT 8 OUNCES
STORAGE: GLASS SPRAY BOTTLE
PREP TIME: 15 MINUTES, PLUS COOLING TIME

Your hair will receive a wealth of benefits from the calendula in this remedy—its regenerative and soothing properties help hair maintain its natural shine and grow stronger at the same.

Scant 1 cup water
1 calendula flower tea bag, or chamomile tea bag
1 tablespoon sea salt
1 teaspoon sweet almond oil
1 tablespoon apple cider vinegar
1 tablespoon freshly squeezed lemon juice
1 teaspoon aloe vera gel
5 drops rosemary essential oil

1. In a small nonreactive saucepan set over high heat, bring the water to a boil.

2. Add the tea bag and steep for 10 minutes. Discard the tea bag.

3. Carefully pour the liquid into a glass spray bottle. Add the sea salt and sweet almond oil. Cover and shake well until dissolved and combined. Cool completely.

4. Add the cider vinegar, lemon juice, aloe vera gel, and rosemary essential oil. Shake to mix well.

5. Shake well before each use. Spray on clean, damp hair.

OILY HAIR

Oily hair doesn't stem solely from a lack of cleanliness. More often, a person's genetic makeup causes an overproduction of oils coming from the sebaceous glands in the scalp. While more frequent shampooing can help to a degree, harsh chemicals in over-the-counter products can lead to brittle and breaking hair follicles. If this sounds like you, try some of these at-home remedies for a change.

LAVENDER SCALP TONER

YIELD: ABOUT 6 OUNCES
STORAGE: SQUEEZE BOTTLE
PREP TIME: 2 MINUTES
TREATMENT TIME: 10 MINUTES

Lavender is one of the sweetest smelling and most versatile essential oils. But feel free to substitute another oil, such as tea tree, cedarwood, lemon, or peppermint, if you prefer.

½ cup water
¼ cup apple cider vinegar
15 to 30 drops lavender essential oil

1. In a squeeze bottle, combine the water, cider vinegar, and lavender essential oil. Cover and shake well.
2. After washing your hair, squirt the liquid onto your scalp until all affected areas are coated.
3. Wring out any excess liquid. Let sit for 10 minutes.
4. Add some conditioner to the hair ends if they feel dry.
5. Towel-dry your hair and style as usual.

CUCUMBER-LEMON CLEANSER

YIELD: 1 TREATMENT
STORAGE: NOT RECOMMENDED
PREP TIME: 5 MINUTES
TREATMENT TIME: 5 MINUTES

Cucumber's cooling properties help diminish dull, greasy hair, while its high silicon and sulfur content promotes hair growth.

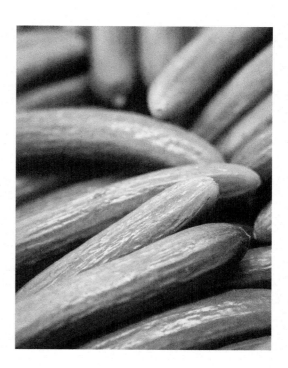

1 cup peeled, diced cucumber

Juice of 1 lemon

1 tablespoon apple cider vinegar

1. In a blender, combine the cucumber, lemon juice, and cider vinegar. Pulse until smooth.

2. Massage into the hair and scalp as you would shampoo. Let sit for up to 5 minutes.

3. Rinse well.

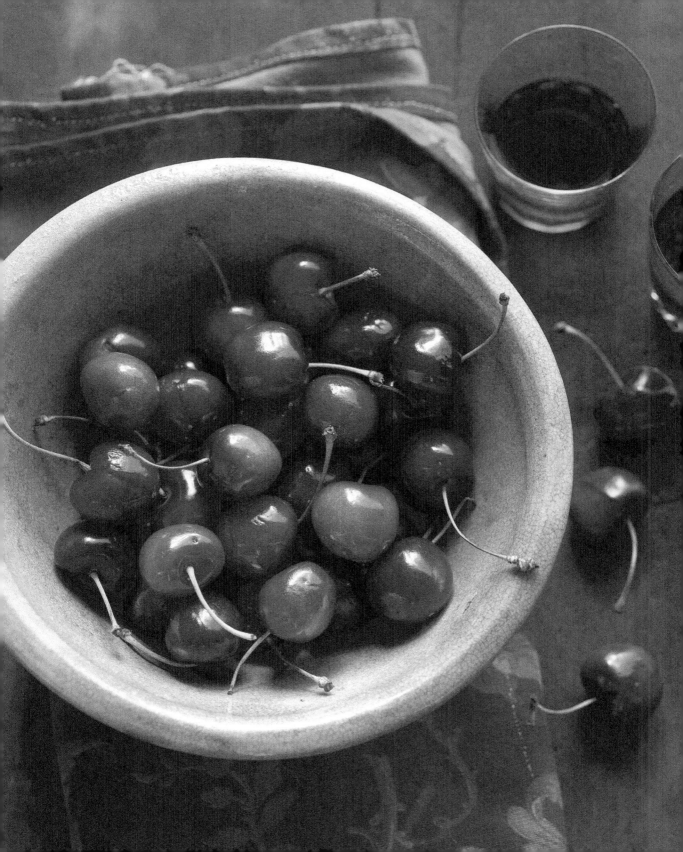

Chapter Five

COMMON AILMENTS

66 Arthritis
Cherry-Apple Cider Nectar
Citrus Joint Juice

68 Cold and Flu
Vinegar Vapor for
Stuffy Sinuses
Fire Cider
Elderberry Shrub
Four Thieves Vinegar

72 Constipation
Psyllium Solution
Tender Tummy Rub
Orange-Coconut
Constipation Chews

74 Cuts, Stings, Bites,
and Scrapes
Plantain Poultice
Black Salve

76 Earache
Essential Earache Rub
Allium Ear Dropper

78 Heartburn and
Indigestion
Peppermint, Ginger, and
Fennel Sipper
Aloe-Lemon Shooter

80 Leg Cramps
Warm Mint Compress
Chocolate Mineral Smoothie

82 Nausea and
Morning Sickness
Ginger Switchel
Fennel Tea

84 Sore Throat
Bone Broth Sipper
Licorice Root Gargle

ARTHRITIS

Some medical professionals believe that a buildup of acid crystals in the joints is what causes arthritis. More accepted is the idea that osteoarthritis is caused by a wearing away of cartilage that lines the joints. Either way, there are anecdotes all over the Internet from arthritis sufferers who swear they have assuaged their joint pain by consuming a little apple cider vinegar each day.

CHERRY-APPLE CIDER NECTAR

YIELD: ABOUT 2½ CUPS
STORAGE: REFRIGERATE IN A GLASS JAR
PREP TIME: 5 MINUTES

Tart cherry juice is loaded with anthocyanins, the plant compound that gives cherries their deep red color. These flavonoids are thought to reduce inflammation and pain in joints and muscles.

1 cup tart cherry juice
1 cup apple cider vinegar

1. In a sealable glass jar, combine the tart cherry juice and cider vinegar. Stir to mix well.

2. To make one serving: In a tall glass, add 2 teaspoons of the mixture and fill with sparkling or still water.

3. Seal the jar and refrigerate the remaining mixture for up to 2 weeks.

CITRUS JOINT JUICE

YIELD: 4 SERVINGS
STORAGE: SEALED GLASS CONTAINER
PREP TIME: 15 MINUTES

Citrus fruits are vitamin-C powerhouses: they help prevent free radical damage in cartilage that leads to inflammatory conditions like arthritis. Known as the relaxation mineral, magnesium citrate is one of the most absorbable forms of this important mineral; you can purchase it in powder form at a health food store.

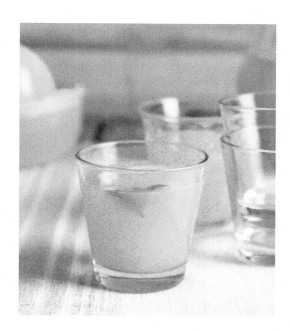

1 grapefruit

1 orange

1 lemon

2 celery stalks

2 tablespoons apple cider vinegar

1 tablespoon magnesium citrate powder

2 cups water

Raw honey, for sweetening (optional)

1. In a juicer, process the grapefruit, orange, lemon, and celery. Discard the pulp.

2. To the juice, stir in the cider vinegar, magnesium citrate powder, and water. Taste and add honey (if using) to reach the desired sweetness.

3. Drink one-fourth of the mixture each morning with breakfast.

4. Seal and refrigerate leftovers for up to 2 weeks.

COLD AND FLU

Fever, chills, respiratory difficulty, and a sore throat are all signs that flu season is headed your way. Don't be a helpless bystander when the aches start. Try a few of these preventive treatments when those around you begin to feel sick. Even if you do end up getting sick, the ingredients in the following recipes are sure to help shorten the length of illness.

VINEGAR VAPOR FOR STUFFY SINUSES

YIELD: 1 TREATMENT
STORAGE: NOT RECOMMENDED
PREP TIME: 5 MINUTES
TREATMENT TIME: 5 TO 10 MINUTES

When breathing gets tough, steam your way to clear sinuses with this potent concoction. Try adding other elements, such as a couple of drops of eucalyptus essential oil or some cardamom pods.

Boiling water, for mixing

2 to 3 tablespoons freshly squeezed lemon juice

2 to 3 tablespoons apple cider vinegar

Handful of fresh mint leaves, torn into pieces

1. Fill a large nonreactive bowl half way with the boiling water.
2. Add the lemon juice, cider vinegar, and mint leaves.
3. Place your face over the bowl, with your head covered by a towel to hold in the steam. Breathe in the steam and aroma for 5 to 10 minutes. End the treatment early if you become too hot or your symptoms are agitated.

FIRE CIDER

YIELD: ABOUT 2 PINTS
STORAGE: REFRIGERATE IN A SEALED GLASS JAR OR
BOTTLE UP TO 1 YEAR
PREP TIME: 20 MINUTES, PLUS 3 TO 6 WEEKS
INFUSING TIME

Many claim that one shot of this traditional cider remedy will cure a cold. Given time to sit and infuse, the blended ingredients will be more effective. This spicy elixir can be taken as a 1-ounce "shot" for adults, or diluted in tea or juice for both adults and children.

½ cup peeled and diced fresh horseradish

½ cup peeled and diced garlic cloves

½ cup peeled and diced onion

½ cup peeled and diced fresh ginger

¼ cup peeled and diced fresh turmeric root

1 habanero chile or jalapeño chile, sliced

1 orange, peeled, quartered, and diced

1 lemon, peeled, quartered, and diced

1 tablespoon black peppercorns

1 tablespoon dried rosemary (optional)

1 tablespoon dried thyme (optional)

4 to 5 cups apple cider vinegar, plus more as needed

¼ cup raw honey

1. In a large lidded glass container, combine the horseradish, garlic, onion, ginger, turmeric, chile, orange, lemon, black peppercorns, rosemary (if using), and thyme (if using).

2. Pour in the cider vinegar until all ingredients are covered. Seal the container with a nonreactive lid. Shake well.

3. Place the container in a dark place. Let sit for 3 to 6 weeks, and shake it daily.

4. Strain the vinegar into a smaller, clean glass jar. Stir in the honey.

5. Seal and refrigerate.

ELDERBERRY SHRUB

YIELD: 1½ CUPS SYRUP
STORAGE: REFRIGERATE IN A SEALED GLASS JAR OR
BOTTLE UP TO 1 YEAR
PREP TIME: 15 MINUTES, PLUS 24 HOURS
REFRIGERATION TIME

*What has more vitamin C than an orange
and contains antiviral properties?
Elderberries! Sambucus, or elder plant, is
a genus of flowering plants whose berries
have been used medicinally for hundreds
of years.*

1 cup fresh elderberries, washed and dried

2 cups apple cider vinegar

1½ cups raw honey

2 tablespoons dried ground ginger

1 teaspoon ground cinnamon

½ teaspoon ground cloves

1. In a nonreactive saucepan, lightly mash the elderberries with a fork. Stir in the cider vinegar. Bring to a boil over medium heat, stirring well. Boil for 5 minutes. Remove from the heat. Cool until lukewarm.

2. Using a fine-mesh strainer, nut milk bag, or cheesecloth, strain the liquid into a glass bowl. Discard the leftover berry flesh.

3. Stir in the honey, ginger, cinnamon, and cloves.

4. Refrigerate in a sealed glass jar or bottle for 24 hours.

5. The preventive dose for a child is ½ to 1 teaspoon per day; for an adult, 1½ teaspoons to 1 tablespoon per day. These servings may also be mixed with sparkling or still water.

Note: Because this recipe contains honey, **it should not be used for children under one year of age**.

FOUR THIEVES VINEGAR

YIELD: 1 QUART
STORAGE: REFRIGERATE IN SEALED GLASS JARS OR
BOTTLES UP TO 1 YEAR
PREP TIME: 5 TO 10 MINUTES, PLUS 6 TO 8 WEEKS
INFUSING TIME

According to legend, in the fourteenth century, four French thieves robbing the dead during the Bubonic Plague survived by drinking this concoction. Today, you can find many recipes for Four Thieves Vinegar. After six weeks, taste it. The longer it brews, the stronger and more potent it becomes.

2 tablespoons dried thyme

2 tablespoons dried rosemary

2 tablespoons dried sage

2 tablespoons dried lavender

2 tablespoons dried mint

2 teaspoons ground cinnamon

2 teaspoons ground cloves

2 teaspoons minced raw garlic

1 (32-ounce) bottle apple cider vinegar

Splash of fresh lemon juice (optional)

1. In a large glass container with a nonreactive lid, combine the thyme, rosemary, sage, lavender, mint, cinnamon, cloves, and garlic. Pour the vinegar over the ingredients. Add the lemon juice (if using).

2. Leave in a cool, dark place for 6 to 8 weeks, shaking daily if possible.

3. When ready, use a fine-mesh sieve to strain out the herbs. Discard the herbs.

4. Transfer the liquid to several smaller glass jars, sealed tightly, for easier storage and access.

5. Drink up: Adults take 1 tablespoon diluted in tea or water; children take 1 teaspoon diluted in tea or water.

CONSTIPATION

You're a likely candidate for constipation if you don't consume enough dietary fiber or drink enough water throughout your day. However, there are other more serious conditions, such as irritable bowel syndrome (IBS), which is defined as a disruption of intestinal movements. Apple cider vinegar has the ability to permeate the intestinal tract and eliminate harmful bacteria, which may be aggravating your body's attempts at proper digestion.

PSYLLIUM SOLUTION

YIELD: 1 SERVING
STORAGE: NOT RECOMMENDED
PREP TIME: 1 MINUTE

Ground psyllium seed husks are an indigestible form of soluble dietary fiber often used to relieve constipation. When combined with water, these husks create a gel-like bulk that pushes through the digestive tract, cleansing the walls of mucus and other toxins present in the colon.

---

1 tablespoon apple cider vinegar
1 tablespoon ground psyllium husks
1½ teaspoons raw honey
1 cup water

1. In a tall glass, stir together the cider vinegar, psyllium husks, honey, and water.
2. Drink all of the solution slowly between meals.

TENDER TUMMY RUB

YIELD: ABOUT 3 TREATMENTS
STORAGE: SMALL GLASS BOTTLE
PREP TIME: 1 MINUTE
TREATMENT TIME: 5 TO 10 MINUTES

Giving yourself an abdominal massage with digestion-stimulating essential oils is a fantastic way to get things moving in your gastrointestinal tract. Here ginger and fennel essential oils combine for this treatment, but other great topical essential oil choices for relieving constipation include orange, tarragon, aniseed, and peppermint.

1 tablespoon apple cider vinegar

1 tablespoon olive oil or avocado oil

5 drops fennel essential oil

5 drops ginger essential oil

1. In a small glass bottle, combine the cider vinegar, olive or avocado oil, fennel essential oil, and ginger essential oil. Cover and shake well.

2. Pour a few drops of the mixture into the palm of your hand. Starting from the lower right side, gently massage your abdomen. This is where your colon should start and begin to ascend. Gently move your hand up toward the bottom of your rib cage and continue to massage in a circular motion down the left side of your abdomen.

Note: The direction specified is very important, since this is the direction your digestion flows.

ORANGE-COCONUT CONSTIPATION CHEWS

YIELD: ABOUT 4 SERVINGS
STORAGE: REFRIGERATE IN A SEALED CONTAINER
PREP TIME: 10 MINUTES, PLUS 1 HOUR FREEZING TIME

Slippery elm powder brings calming relief from numerous intestinal problems, including constipation. It creates a slimy film that soothes pain caused by irritable bowel syndrome, colitis, or constipation. It is also high in fiber and, therefore, moves through the intestines, absorbing toxins and creating bulk as it soaks up fluids.

1 tablespoon apple cider vinegar

1 cup coconut oil, melted

1 teaspoon slippery elm powder

¼ cup orange juice

3 tablespoons raw honey

½ teaspoon sea salt

1. Place a silicone candy mold tray in the freezer for at least 10 minutes. (This will help the finished product set better without separating the ingredients.)

2. In a medium nonreactive bowl, whisk together all the ingredients. Or, for a more thorough blend, use a small food processor or blender.

3. Fill each chilled candy mold with batter. Freeze for 1 hour, or until the chews can be removed in one piece.

4. Dosage for children is two chews. For adults, it's four.

5. Store in an airtight glass jar in the refrigerator for up to 1 week.

CUTS, STINGS, BITES, AND SCRAPES

On some jellyfish-infested beaches, vinegar is kept stocked at the lifeguard towers for easy access to this quick remedy. Apple cider vinegar acts as an effective antiseptic for many types of aquatic stings like jellyfish or fire coral.

PLANTAIN POULTICE

YIELD: 1 CUP
STORAGE: GLASS JAR
PREP TIME: 10 MINUTES (OR 30 TO 40 MINUTES IF USING DRIED PLANTAIN LEAF)

Plantain leaf is a common weed you may have growing in your backyard. If not, you can buy it online (see Resources, page 201). The compounds in plantain leaf are believed to relieve skin irritation and act as a mild expectorant, drawing out toxins.

¼ cup apple cider vinegar

¼ cup water

½ cup dried plantain leaf

10 to 15 drops of any combination of the following essential oils: thyme, tea tree, lemongrass, clove, rosemary, lemon, lavender, and eucalyptus

1. In a food processor or blender, combine the cider vinegar, water, and plantain leaf. If using dried plantain leaf, soak it in the liquid for 20 to 30 minutes before blending. Pulse until a thin paste forms. Transfer to a glass storage jar.

2. Add the essential oils of your choice. Stir well to combine.

3. Apply a thin layer to affected areas, and cover with a small bandage.

4. Store the remaining paste in an airtight glass jar for up to 1 year.

BLACK SALVE

YIELD: ABOUT 5½ OUNCES
STORAGE: GLASS JAR
PREP TIME: 10 MINUTES, PLUS COOLING TIME

Beeswax is a natural skin protectant, keeping unwanted matter out while allowing the skin to breathe. The activated charcoal and clay in this recipe work together beautifully to draw out unwanted toxins from the skin, whether it's insect poison causing an itch or jellyfish toxins causing a painful sting.

¼ cup coconut oil

2 teaspoons beeswax

¼ cup castor oil

2 teaspoons (about 10 capsules) activated charcoal

4 teaspoons bentonite clay

15 drops lavender essential oil

15 drops tea tree oil

1 tablespoon apple cider vinegar

1. In a medium glass jar, combine the coconut oil and beeswax.

2. Place the jar in a small saucepan of water set over low heat. Melt the ingredients in the jar, and stir to combine.

3. To the jar, add the castor oil, activated charcoal, bentonite clay, lavender essential oil, and tea tree oil. Stir to combine. Let cool until it becomes a spreadable salve.

4. Splash the infected area with the apple cider vinegar. Let it air-dry.

5. Apply a small amount of the salve to the injured area and cover with a small bandage.

6. Reapply and rebandage every 3 to 6 hours.

7. Store the remaining salve in an airtight glass jar in a cool, dry place for up to 1 year.

EARACHE

Recurring ear infections in children are all too common today, and are often followed by a round of tubes, a surgical procedure that implants plastic tubing that helps clear fluid from the middle ear into the ear canal. Antibiotics are not always the answer and can often cause greater problems down the road. Many earaches and infections can be cleared up quickly using natural support.

ESSENTIAL EARACHE RUB

YIELD: 2 TEASPOONS / 10 ML
STORAGE: GLASS ROLLERBALL BOTTLE
PREP TIME: 5 MINUTES

Never put essential oils inside the ear canal. Rubbing them around the outside of the ear, however, encourages proper drainage and circulation, and promotes healing.

---

1 teaspoon apple cider vinegar

1 teaspoon castor oil

5 to 7 drops lavender essential oil

5 to 7 drops tea tree essential oil

1. In a glass rollerball bottle, combine the cider vinegar, castor oil, lavender essential oil, and tea tree essential oil. Cover and shake well.

2. Use the rollerball to apply the liquid around the outside of the ear, focusing on behind the ear canal and down toward the neck. Continue to rub in with your fingers, working the mixture downward to facilitate proper drainage.

3. Store remaining treatment in the same glass rollerball bottle, in a cool, dark place, for up to 6 months.

ALLIUM EAR DROPPER

YIELD: ABOUT 2 TEASPOONS / 10 ML
STORAGE: 10 ML GLASS DROPPER BOTTLE
PREP TIME: 10 MINUTES
TREATMENT TIME: 5 TO 10 MINUTES

Rubbing alcohol is used in this remedy instead of water to promote removal of moisture from the ear canal, which can foster bacteria growth that causes infection. Alliums are bulbous plants from the onion genus, such as garlic, leeks, and chives, typically containing antimicrobial properties.

For the garlic, or onion, juice
2 or 3 garlic cloves, peeled, or ½ small onion peeled and cut into chunks

For the allium ear dropper mixture
1 teaspoon rubbing alcohol
1 teaspoon apple cider vinegar

To make the garlic, or onion, juice

1. Press the garlic cloves, or onion chunks, through a garlic press. Alternately, put either in a small food processor or blender and pulse to produce a wet mush.

2. Over a small bowl, press the solids into a fine-mesh sieve to extract the juice. You need about 10 drops of juice.

To make the allium ear dropper mixture

In a glass dropper bottle, combine 10 drops of garlic juice, or onion juice, the rubbing alcohol, and cider vinegar. Cover and shake well.

To administer

1. Use the dropper to wet a clean cotton ball (15 to 20 drops). Have the person lie down, with the head turned so the affected ear faces up. Gently place the cotton ball in the ear opening and leave for 5 to 10 minutes.

2. Discard the cotton ball. Have the person tilt their head to the side opposite the affected ear to drain out any remaining fluid.

HEARTBURN AND INDIGESTION

Acidic is the natural and proper state of the stomach. So, in many cases of supposed heartburn, too much stomach acid is not actually the culprit. More often than not, heartburn and indigestion symptoms are caused by not having enough stomach acid, which causes it to churn violently in order to make the best of what it does have. Apple cider vinegar has been used for centuries to encourage proper digestion and stomach acid secretion.

PEPPERMINT, GINGER, AND FENNEL SIPPER

YIELD: 1 SERVING
STORAGE: NOT RECOMMENDED
PREP TIME: 2 MINUTES

Fennel seeds contain an organic compound called anethole, which has become known as a gastrointestinal antispasmodic. For relief similar to what this remedy provides, you can also just chew fennel seeds.

8 ounces water
1 tablespoon apple cider vinegar
1 drop food-grade peppermint essential oil
1 drop food-grade ginger essential oil
1 drop food-grade fennel essential oil

1. In a tall glass, combine the water, cider vinegar, peppermint essential oil, ginger essential oil, and fennel essential oil. Stir well.

2. Sip between meals for relief.

ALOE-LEMON SHOOTER

YIELD: 1 SHOT
STORAGE: NOT RECOMMENDED
PREP TIME: 2 MINUTES

While lemons contain citric acid, they actually leave a soothing alkaline residue in the body when consumed, making them an easy and great choice for relieving and soothing acid reflux–like symptoms.

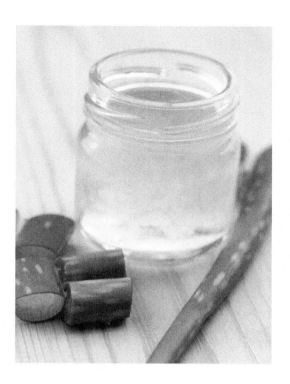

3 tablespoons aloe vera juice
1 teaspoon apple cider vinegar
Juice of 1 lemon

1. In a small glass, stir together the aloe vera juice, cider vinegar, and lemon juice.

2. Drink 10 to 20 minutes before a meal.

LEG CRAMPS

Leg cramps, especially nocturnal ones, can plague anyone. Younger children can get them in the form of "growing pains," while adults often cramp up in reaction to a mineral deficiency or poor circulation resulting from sitting at a desk all day.

WARM MINT COMPRESS

YIELD: 1 TREATMENT
STORAGE: NOT RECOMMENDED
PREP TIME: 5 MINUTES
TREATMENT TIME: 20 MINUTES

Ease sore legs and strained muscles. Wrap your limbs in warm cloths soaked with apple cider vinegar and plant oils like clove, wintergreen, and peppermint that possess warming, anesthetic properties.

---

1 cup apple cider vinegar
5 to 6 drops wintergreen essential oil
5 to 6 drops peppermint essential oil
5 to 6 drops clove essential oil

1. In a small nonreactive saucepan set over low heat, warm the cider vinegar.
2. Add the wintergreen essential oil, peppermint essential oil, and clove essential oil, and stir to combine.
3. Dampen two clean cloths, each large enough to wrap around one leg, with water.
4. Soak each cloth in half of the compress solution.
5. Wrap each leg in one of the wet cloths and rest for 20 minutes.

CHOCOLATE MINERAL SMOOTHIE

YIELD: 2 SERVINGS
STORAGE: REFRIGERATE IN A SEALED GLASS JAR
PREP TIME: 6 MINUTES

Leg cramps, especially nocturnal ones, can be a sign that you need more minerals in your diet, like magnesium, calcium, and potassium. In this remedy, the almond milk provides calcium. The cocoa powder and spinach are rich in magnesium and other trace minerals. The bananas, avocado, and yogurt provide potassium.

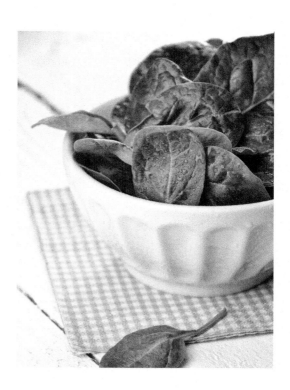

1 cup almond milk

½ cup full-fat yogurt

1 banana

1 cup fresh spinach

½ avocado

2 tablespoons cocoa powder

1 tablespoon apple cider vinegar

¼ teaspoon sea salt

1 tablespoon raw honey (optional)

Water, to thin, as needed

1. In the blender, layer the almond milk, yogurt, banana, spinach, avocado, cocoa powder, cider vinegar, sea salt, and honey (if using).

2. Blend on high until completely smooth. Thin with a little bit of water, if necessary.

3. Pour into two glasses and serve.

NAUSEA AND MORNING SICKNESS

Whether it's a new pregnancy or a windy road trip that's caused it, nausea is no fun for anyone. When our stomachs refuse to settle, it's hard to get the proper nutrients into our bodies. These remedies don't require any chewing though—just sip on them when nausea strikes.

GINGER SWITCHEL

YIELD: 2 SERVINGS
STORAGE: REFRIGERATE IN A SEALED GLASS JAR UP TO 1 WEEK
PREP TIME: 20 MINUTES, PLUS COOLING TIME

In the 1800s, switchel was a thirst quencher for overheated harvest laborers. Ginger and vinegar lessen the nausea brought on by drinking plain cold water on an empty stomach. Today, ginger has become renowned as a safer alternative to antinausea drugs. For a mellower flavor, use dried, ground ginger.

4 cups water, divided
2 tablespoons minced fresh peeled ginger
¼ cup freshly squeezed lemon juice
2 tablespoons raw honey or maple syrup
2 tablespoons apple cider vinegar

1. In a small saucepan set over high heat, bring 1 cup of the water to a boil.

2. Add the ginger. Boil for 2 minutes. Remove from the heat, cover, and infuse for 15 minutes.

3. Into a large glass jar, strain the mixture through a fine-mesh sieve. Discard the ginger flesh. Refrigerate the ginger infusion until well chilled.

4. Stir in the lemon juice, honey, cider vinegar, and the remaining 3 cups water.

5. Pour into two glasses and serve.

FENNEL TEA

YIELD: 1 SERVING
STORAGE: NOT RECOMMENDED
PREP TIME: 5 TO 10 MINUTES

Fennel seeds, which are actually the plant's fruit and not a true seed, are popular in Indian cuisine, where they're traditionally chewed after a meal to prevent indigestion.

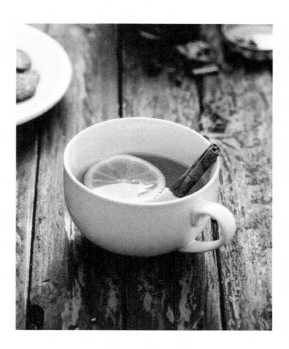

2 cups water

1 tablespoon fennel seeds

1 cinnamon stick

1 tablespoon apple cider vinegar

Raw honey, to sweeten

1. In a small nonreactive saucepan set over high heat, bring the water to a boil. Remove from the heat.

2. Add the fennel seeds and cinnamon stick and steep for 5 to 10 minutes. Cool slightly.

3. Stir in the cider vinegar and honey.

4. Sip throughout the morning, or whenever nausea persists.

SORE THROAT

See a tinge of bright red at the back of your throat? This means inflammation is on the rise and pain is just around the corner—if you aren't experiencing some swallowing discomfort already. Killing germs and soothing inflammation are key to fighting the common sore throat. Thankfully, with the help of a few kitchen cupboard friends, apple cider vinegar can do both!

BONE BROTH SIPPER

YIELD: 1 SERVING
STORAGE: SEALED GLASS JAR
TIME: 5 MINUTES

Chicken soup is good for the soul . . . and a sore throat. Enhance the healing properties of the broth with a little apple cider vinegar. Sip it from a mug as you would tea, and feel the soothing warmth.

---

2 cups Homemade Chicken Stock (page 139)
1 garlic clove, crushed
1 tablespoon apple cider vinegar
¼ teaspoon hot pepper sauce

1. In a small saucepan set over medium heat, warm the broth until just before boiling. Remove from the heat and transfer to a mug.

2. Stir in the garlic, cider vinegar, and hot sauce. Sip the mixture for sore throat relief.

Note: The garlic should sink to the bottom and stay there, but if not, strain it out and discard.

LICORICE ROOT GARGLE

YIELD: 1 SERVING
STORAGE: SEALED GLASS JAR
PREP TIME: 10 MINUTES
TREATMENT TIME: 1 MINUTE

The anti-inflammatory properties of licorice root soothe the mucous membranes in your throat and also reduce swelling. It's a natural demulcent, which means it relieves irritation by forming a protective film. Licorice root is not recommended for use by pregnant women.

1 cup very warm water

2 tablespoons dried, chopped licorice root

1 tablespoon apple cider vinegar

1 tablespoon raw honey

¼ teaspoon ground cinnamon

¼ teaspoon sea salt

1. In a small saucepan set over high heat, bring the water to a boil.

2. Add the licorice root and boil for 2 minutes. Remove from the heat. Pour through a fine-mesh sieve into a nonreactive container to strain out the licorice root pieces.

3. Stir in the cider vinegar, honey, cinnamon, and sea salt. Allow to cool until lukewarm.

4. Gargle with the warm liquid for 20 seconds to 1 minute, so it gets into the back of your throat. Spit the liquid into a sink when done—do not swallow. Continue with the remaining liquid, as needed, for relief.

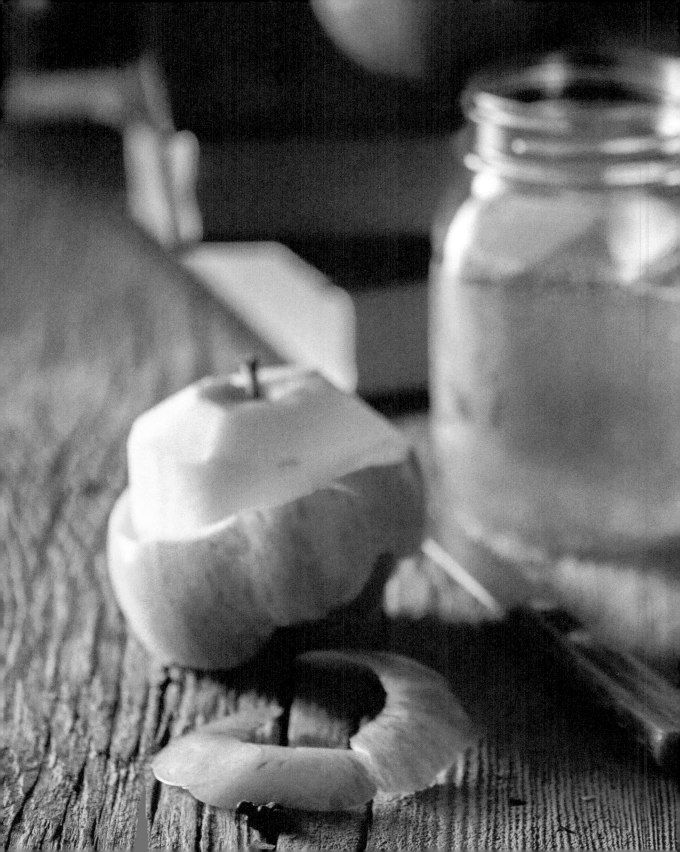

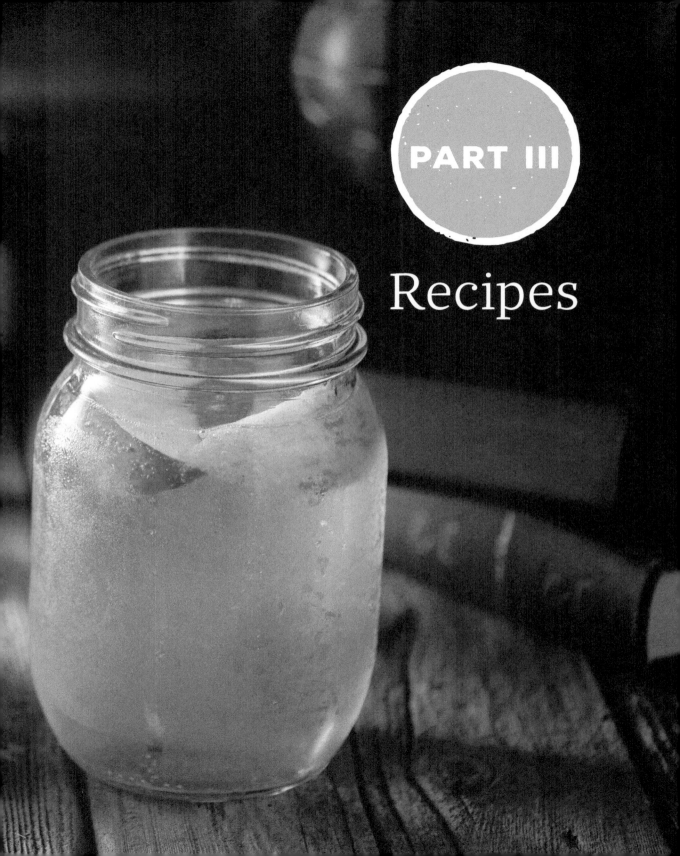

PART III

Recipes

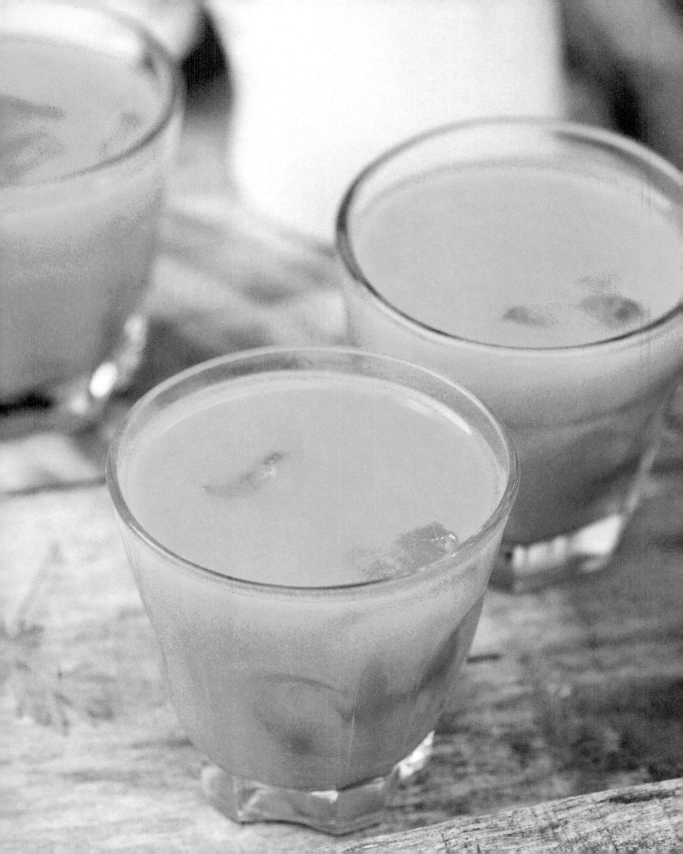

Chapter Six

DRINKS & SMOOTHIES

90   Raspberry Lemonade

91   Citrus Refresher

92   Apple Pie Drink

93   Honey-Lemon Tea

94   Lime-Cider Soda

96   Almond-Berry Smoothie

97   Mango-Ginger Smoothie

98   Tropical Cider Smoothie

99   PB and J Smoothie

101   Pear Green Smoothie

102   Gazpacho Smoothie

103   Bright Carrot Smoothie

104   Avocado-Herb Smoothie

105   Banana-Berry Smoothie

106   Creamy Peach Smoothie

RASPBERRY LEMONADE

GLUTEN FREE **PALEO FRIENDLY** **QUICK & EASY** **VEGAN** VEGETARIAN

SERVES 2 • PREP TIME: 5 MINUTES, PLUS 3 HOURS INFUSING TIME

The cool tartness of perfectly balanced lemonade can cut through the muggiest days of summer. Apple cider vinegar enhances and intensifies the sweetness of the raspberries and the tart lemon flavor in this refreshing beverage. Substitute frozen raspberries for fresh if you can't find quality berries at the market.

---

2 cups water

1 cup freshly squeezed lemon juice

⅓ cup apple cider vinegar

1 tablespoon honey

1 cup fresh raspberries

4 ice cubes

1. In a medium nonreactive bowl, stir together the water, lemon juice, cider vinegar, and honey until well blended.

2. Stir in the raspberries. Cover the bowl.

3. Refrigerate for 3 hours to infuse the liquid.

4. Divide the ice cubes between 2 tall glasses. Pour the raspberry lemonade over the ice and serve.

 TIP Raspberries may be an important addition to obesity management and weight loss because of the phytonutrients, such as rheosmin, found in this colorful berry. Rheosmin might help limit fat absorption by impeding the action of pancreatic lipase, which is a fat-digesting enzyme released by the pancreas.

PER SERVING CALORIES: 103; FAT: 1G; SATURATED FAT: 1G; PROTEIN: 2G; CARBS: 19G; SODIUM: 28MG; FIBER: 5G; SUGAR: 14G

CITRUS REFRESHER

GLUTEN FREE **PALEO FRIENDLY** QUICK & EASY **VEGAN** VEGETARIAN

SERVES 2 • PREP TIME: 5 MINUTES

Red and orange fruit combine to create a sunset-hued drink with triple citrus impact and a hint of sweetness. Ruby red grapefruit was the first grapefruit to be granted a US patent. This glorious fruit is rich in the antioxidant lycopene, which gives it the distinctive ruby color.

2 cups ruby red grapefruit juice

1 cup orange juice

Juice of 1 lime

2 tablespoons apple cider vinegar

2 tablespoons honey

1. In a medium nonreactive bowl, stir together the grapefruit juice, orange juice, lime juice, cider vinegar, and honey.

2. Pour into 2 tall glasses and serve.

PER SERVING CALORIES: 202; FAT: 0G; SATURATED FAT: 0G; PROTEIN: 2G; CARBS: 51G; SODIUM: 3MG; FIBER: 3G; SUGAR: 44G

APPLE PIE DRINK

GLUTEN FREE **PALEO FRIENDLY QUICK & EASY VEGAN** VEGETARIAN

SERVES 2 • PREP TIME: 5 MINUTES

You can whip up this warmly spiced drink quickly when you need an energy lift. Adding apple chunks and ice while blending the ingredients can change this simple drink into a thick smoothie. Tart apples such as McIntosh or Granny Smith are nice additions to this flavor profile.

---

1 cup unsweetened apple juice

¼ cup water

¼ cup apple cider vinegar

2 tablespoons honey

¼ teaspoon ground cinnamon

Pinch of ground cloves

4 ice cubes

1. In a medium nonreactive bowl, stir together the apple juice, water, cider vinegar, honey, cinnamon, and cloves until well blended.

2. Divide the ice cubes between 2 tall glasses. Pour the drink over the ice and serve.

PER SERVING CALORIES: 130; FAT: 0G; SATURATED FAT: 0G; PROTEIN: 0G; CARBS: 32G; SODIUM: 7MG; FIBER: 0G; SUGAR: 31G

HONEY-LEMON TEA

GLUTEN FREE **PALEO FRIENDLY** QUICK & EASY **VEGAN** VEGETARIAN

SERVES 2 • PREP TIME: 5 MINUTES

Many diets and healthy eating plans recommend drinking warm lemon water with honey as the perfect way to start the day. This jazzed-up version aids digestion and provides important electrolytes to hydrate your body. Honey-lemon tea also helps detoxify the liver, boost immunity, and reduce joint pain.

2 cups boiling water, divided

4 tablespoons apple cider vinegar, divided

4 tablespoons freshly squeezed
lemon juice, divided

2 tablespoons honey, divided

¼ teaspoon ground cinnamon, divided

1. Pour the boiling water into 2 mugs.

2. To each of the 2 mugs, add 2 tablespoons cider vinegar, 2 tablespoons lemon juice, 1 tablespoon honey, and ⅛ teaspoon cinnamon. Stir to blend.

3. Serve hot.

PER SERVING CALORIES: 75; FAT: 0G; SATURATED FAT: 0G;
PROTEIN: 0G; CARBS: 18G; SODIUM: 5MG; FIBER: 0G; SUGAR: 18G

LIME-CIDER SODA

GLUTEN FREE **PALEO FRIENDLY QUICK & EASY VEGAN** VEGETARIAN

SERVES 2 • PREP TIME: 5 MINUTES

Sugary, additive-packed soda is not a good choice for quenching thirst or hydrating the body. This tart, slightly spicy soda will hit the spot when you crave a bubbly beverage. Try orange juice, lemon juice, or grapefruit juice instead of lime for different flavors.

2 cups club soda, divided

Juice of 2 limes, divided

2 tablespoons apple cider vinegar, divided

2 tablespoons honey, divided

½ teaspoon ground ginger, divided

Pinch of nutmeg, divided

4 ice cubes, divided

2 fresh mint sprigs

1. In each of 2 tall glasses, combine 1 cup club soda, juice of 1 lime, 1 tablespoon cider vinegar, 1 tablespoon honey, ¼ teaspoon ginger, small pinch of nutmeg, and 2 ice cubes. Stir to blend.

2. Garnish each beverage with 1 mint sprig and serve.

 TIP Club soda contains no calories, carbs, protein, or fat, but this fizzy beverage does contain sodium, which is why it tastes slightly salty. If you are watching your sodium intake for health reasons, use seltzer water instead for all the bubbles and none of the sodium.

PER SERVING CALORIES: 79; FAT: 0G; SATURATED FAT: 0G; PROTEIN: 0G; CARBS: 22G; SODIUM: 52MG; FIBER: 0G; SUGAR: 18G

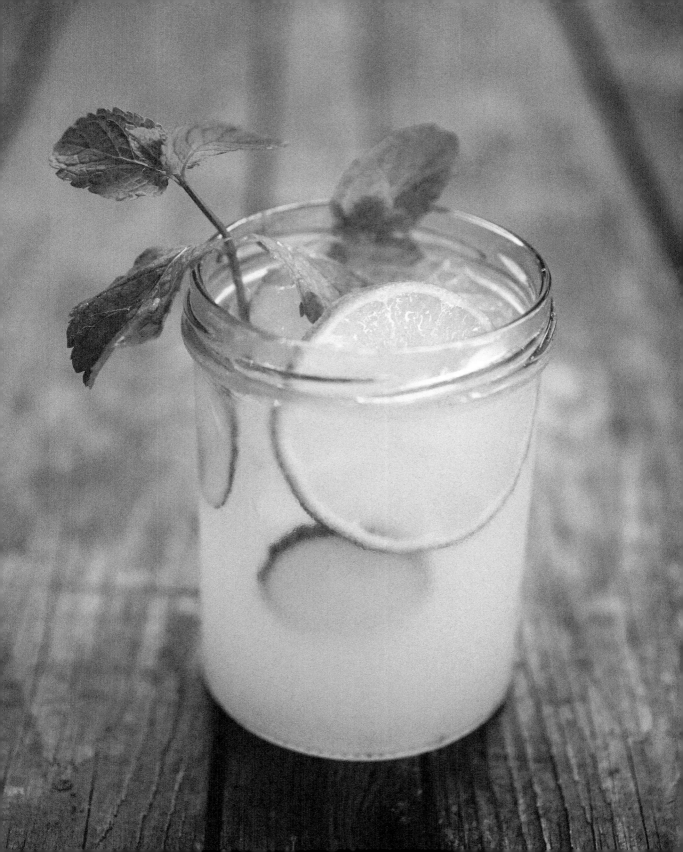

ALMOND-BERRY SMOOTHIE

GLUTEN FREE **PALEO FRIENDLY** QUICK & EASY **VEGAN** VEGETARIAN

SERVES 2 • PREP TIME: 10 MINUTES

Almond milk is a popular choice for many people who do not consume dairy products or soy, making up about 66 percent of the plant-based milk market in the United States. Since almond milk contains only 60 calories per cup with no saturated fat, it is a healthy choice for weight loss. Almond milk is also low in carbs, which means it does not negatively impact blood sugar.

1 banana

½ cup stemmed and shredded kale

½ cup sliced fresh strawberries

½ cup fresh raspberries

1 cup almond milk

2 tablespoons apple cider vinegar

2 tablespoons honey

4 ice cubes

1. In a blender, combine the banana, kale, strawberries, raspberries, almond milk, cider vinegar, and honey. Blend until smooth.

2. Add the ice and blend until thick and smooth.

3. Pour into 2 tall glasses and serve.

PER SERVING CALORIES: 180; FAT: 2G; SATURATED FAT: 0G; PROTEIN: 2G; CARBS: 42G; SODIUM: 73MG; FIBER: 5G; SUGAR: 31G

MANGO-GINGER SMOOTHIE

GLUTEN FREE **PALEO FRIENDLY** QUICK & EASY **VEGAN** VEGETARIAN

SERVES 2 • PREP TIME: 15 MINUTES, PLUS 30 MINUTES SOAKING TIME

The thick texture of this smoothie is enhanced with the addition of chia seeds. Chia seeds have a unique gelling action that helps you feel fuller longer and controls blood sugar spikes. These humble little seeds absorb the flavors of whatever they are soaked in along with nine to twelve times their volume in liquid. Chia seeds contain more omega-3 oil than salmon and are a complete protein.

1 cup almond milk, divided

2 tablespoons chia seeds

1 mango, peeled and pitted

1 banana

½ cup stemmed and shredded kale

½ cup sliced fresh strawberries

3 tablespoons apple cider vinegar

2 teaspoons grated peeled fresh ginger

4 ice cubes

1. In a small bowl, stir together ½ cup of the almond milk and the chia seeds. Set aside to soak for 30 minutes.

2. In a blender, combine the mango, banana, kale, strawberries, cider vinegar, ginger, and remaining ½ cup almond milk. Add the chia seeds and their liquid. Blend until very smooth.

3. Add the ice cubes and blend until thick and smooth.

4. Pour into 2 tall glasses and serve.

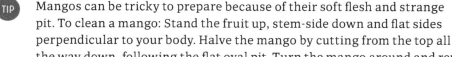 **TIP** Mangos can be tricky to prepare because of their soft flesh and strange pit. To clean a mango: Stand the fruit up, stem-side down and flat sides perpendicular to your body. Halve the mango by cutting from the top all the way down, following the flat oval pit. Turn the mango around and repeat on the other side. Separate the halves. Make lengthwise and crosswise cuts in each mango half, taking care not to cut through the skin. Then turn the mango halves inside out so that the cut sections protrude. Cut the sections off, or remove them with your fingers, close to the peel.

PER SERVING CALORIES: 200; FAT: 4G; SATURATED FAT: 0G;
PROTEIN: 4G; CARBS: 41G; SODIUM: 102MG; FIBER: 7G; SUGAR: 25G

TROPICAL CIDER SMOOTHIE

GLUTEN FREE **PALEO FRIENDLY** QUICK & EASY **VEGAN** VEGETARIAN

SERVES 2 • PREP TIME: 5 MINUTES

The combination of pineapple and banana will spirit you away to visions of white sand beaches and azure waters. Fresh ripe pineapple provides the best flavor, but canned unsweetened fruit in juice is an acceptable substitute. When picking the pineapple, make sure the fruit has a sweet fragrance and yellow skin because pineapple does not continue to ripen after it's picked.

1½ cups unsweetened coconut milk

1 cup fresh pineapple chunks

1 frozen banana, sliced

2 tablespoons apple cider vinegar

1 teaspoon vanilla extract

1 teaspoon unsweetened shredded coconut, divided

1. In a blender, combine the coconut milk, pineapple, banana, cider vinegar, and vanilla. Blend until smooth.

2. Pour into 2 tall glasses. Top each with ½ teaspoon of the coconut and serve.

PER SERVING CALORIES: 139; FAT: 4G; SATURATED FAT: 3G; PROTEIN: 1G; CARBS: 26G; SODIUM: 3MG; FIBER: 4G; SUGAR: 16G

PB AND J SMOOTHIE

GLUTEN FREE **QUICK & EASY VEGAN VEGETARIAN**

SERVES 2 • PREP TIME: 5 MINUTES

Peanut butter and jam are a legendary combination for sandwiches and other dishes, so this smoothie will have a familiar flavor. The apple cider vinegar and natural peanut butter prevent this drink from being too sweet and the flaxseed adds interesting texture. Substitute sesame seeds for the flaxseed if you want a toastier taste.

1½ cups almond milk, plus additional as needed

1 frozen banana, sliced

1 cup frozen strawberries

¼ cup natural peanut butter

2 tablespoons honey

1 tablespoon ground flaxseed

1 tablespoon apple cider vinegar

1. In a blender, combine the almond milk, banana, strawberries, peanut butter, honey, flaxseed, and cider vinegar. Blend until smooth, adding more almond milk, if necessary, to achieve the desired thickness.

2. Pour into 2 tall glasses and serve.

 TIP If you are not familiar with natural peanut butter, the separation of oil and solids can be a little unexpected. Conventional peanut butter often has vegetable oil added to stabilize the texture and prevent the separation found in natural products. Simply stir natural peanut butter before using it to ensure even oil distribution and texture.

PER SERVING CALORIES: 384; FAT: 19G; SATURATED FAT: 3G; PROTEIN: 12G; CARBS: 44G; SODIUM: 145MG; FIBER: 7G; SUGAR: 31G

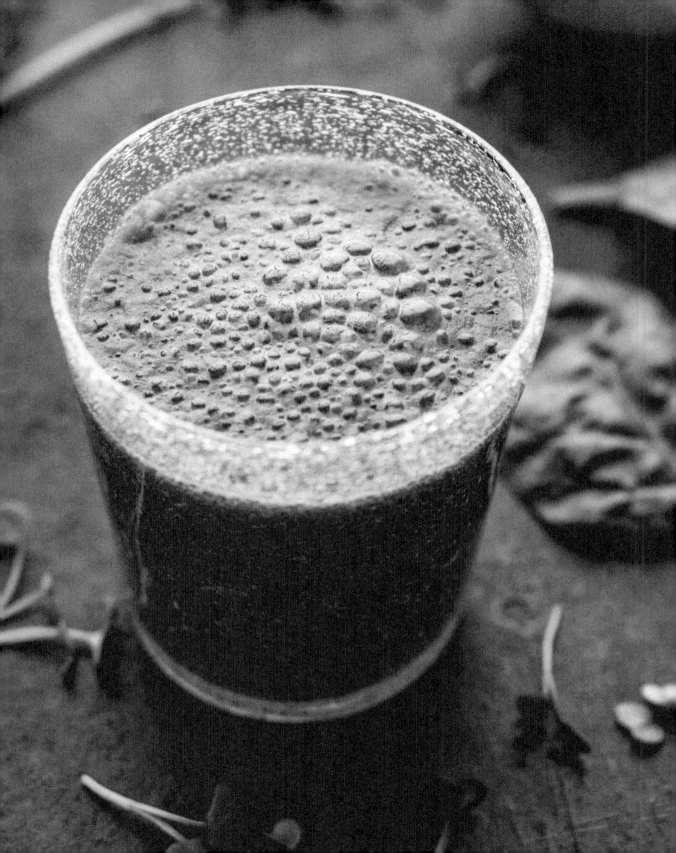

PEAR GREEN SMOOTHIE

GLUTEN FREE **PALEO FRIENDLY** QUICK & EASY **VEGAN** VEGETARIAN

SERVES 2 • PREP TIME: 10 MINUTES

Green smoothies are popular with fitness and weightlifting enthusiasts, as well as anyone trying to eat healthier or lose weight. Dark leafy greens, such as spinach, are superfoods packed with phytonutrients, chlorophyll, vitamins, and minerals. You can also use kale, beet greens, arugula, or Swiss chard in this recipe.

---

2 cups fresh baby spinach

1 ripe pear, cored and chopped

1 cup unsweetened apple juice

2 tablespoons unsalted shelled sunflower seeds

2 tablespoons apple cider vinegar

½ teaspoon ground cinnamon

½ teaspoon ground nutmeg

4 ice cubes

1. In a blender, combine the spinach, pear, apple juice, sunflower seeds, cider vinegar, cinnamon, and nutmeg. Blend until smooth.

2. Add the ice and blend until thick and smooth.

3. Pour into 2 tall glasses and serve.

 TIP   Raw sunflower seeds work nicely in this smoothie, but for a richer taste, try roasted, unsalted seeds. You can roast the seeds yourself in a 300°F oven for 10 to 15 minutes.

PER SERVING CALORIES: 130; FAT: 2G; SATURATED FAT: 0G; PROTEIN: 2G; CARBS: 28G; SODIUM: 29MG; FIBER: 4G; SUGAR: 21G

GAZPACHO SMOOTHIE

GLUTEN FREE **PALEO FRIENDLY QUICK & EASY VEGAN** VEGETARIAN

SERVES 2 • PREP TIME: 10 MINUTES

Check the label carefully on tomato juice before purchasing to weed out products astronomically high in sodium. Commercial vegetable juices often have added salt and flavorings, which can add up to 400mg of sodium or more per cup. Look for reduced-sodium products, or juice your own tomatoes for this smoothie.

1 cup tomato juice

1 tomato, cut into wedges

½ English cucumber, sliced

3 tablespoons apple cider vinegar

2 tablespoons freshly squeezed lime juice

1 tablespoon chopped fresh cilantro

¼ teaspoon hot sauce

3 ice cubes

1. In a blender, combine the tomato juice, tomato, cucumber, cider vinegar, lime juice, cilantro, and hot sauce. Blend until smooth.

2. Add the ice and blend until thick and smooth.

3. Pour into 2 tall glasses and serve.

 TIP Smoothies are usually meant to be, well, smooth, of course. But this beverage is also lovely left with a bit of texture. Pulse the ingredients instead of blending them and omit the ice cubes for a smoothie that drinks like real gazpacho soup.

PER SERVING CALORIES: 53; FAT: 0G; SATURATED FAT: 0G; PROTEIN: 2G; CARBS: 13G; SODIUM: 348MG; FIBER: 1G; SUGAR: 7G

BRIGHT CARROT SMOOTHIE

GLUTEN FREE **PALEO FRIENDLY** QUICK & EASY **VEGAN** VEGETARIAN

SERVES 2 • PREP TIME: 10 MINUTES

The texture of this smoothie will not necessarily be smooth, because you're blending raw carrots. It is almost impossible to completely purée hard vegetables. If you enjoy the velvety texture of traditional smoothies, lightly blanch or steam the carrots until tender before using them in this recipe.

2 large carrots, peeled and sliced

1 pear, cored and cut into chunks

¾ cup unsweetened apple juice

¼ cup apple cider vinegar

1 teaspoon honey

Juice of 1 lime

¼ teaspoon chopped fresh thyme

4 ice cubes

1. In a blender, combine the carrots, pear, apple juice, cider vinegar, honey, lime juice, and thyme. Blend until smooth.

2. Add the ice cubes and blend until thick and smooth.

3. Pour the mixture into 2 tall glasses and serve.

PER SERVING CALORIES: 131; FAT: 0G; SATURATED FAT: 0G; PROTEIN: 1G; CARBS: 32G; SODIUM: 55MG; FIBER: 4G; SUGAR: 24G

AVOCADO-HERB SMOOTHIE

GLUTEN FREE **PALEO FRIENDLY** QUICK & EASY **VEGAN** VEGETARIAN

SERVES 2 • PREP TIME: 5 MINUTES

Fresh herbs are essential for the color and taste of this drink. Dried herbs lose precious essential oils and usually dull in color when moisture is removed. Any combination of fresh herbs can be blended with avocado, such as oregano, savory, basil, tarragon, and marjoram.

---

1 cup fresh spinach

½ avocado, cubed

1 cup unsweetened apple juice

2 tablespoons apple cider vinegar

1 tablespoon honey

1 tablespoon chopped fresh mint

1 tablespoon chopped fresh parsley

1 tablespoon grated peeled fresh ginger

1. In a blender, combine the spinach, avocado, apple juice, cider vinegar, honey, mint, parsley, and ginger. Blend until very smooth.

2. Pour into 2 tall glasses and serve.

 TIP Leftover avocado can become brown and mushy along the cut edge very quickly, which makes the fruit unsuitable for other uses. To prevent this, place the avocado half in a sealed container with a piece of cut onion. The sulfur in the onion keeps the avocado from oxidizing.

PER SERVING CALORIES: 211; FAT: 10G; SATURATED FAT: 2G; PROTEIN: 2G; CARBS: 30G; SODIUM: 23MG; FIBER: 4G; SUGAR: 23G

BANANA-BERRY SMOOTHIE

GLUTEN FREE **QUICK & EASY** VEGETARIAN

SERVES 2 • PREP TIME: 5 MINUTES

Breakfast has never been easier than whipping together berries, banana, and refreshing cucumber for a satisfying start to the day. English cucumber has a tender, sweet skin that does not need to be removed before blending. Regular cucumbers do need to be peeled before using them in this smoothie because the skin can be bitter, thick, and wax coated.

½ cup sliced fresh strawberries

½ cup fresh blueberries

1 frozen banana, sliced

1 cup whole milk

½ English cucumber

2 tablespoons apple cider vinegar

Pinch of ground cloves

1. In a blender, combine the strawberries, blueberries, banana, milk, cucumber, cider vinegar, and cloves. Blend until smooth.

2. Pour into 2 tall glasses and serve.

PER SERVING CALORIES: 172; FAT: 5G; SATURATED FAT: 2G;
PROTEIN: 6G; CARBS: 30G; SODIUM: 52MG; FIBER: 4G; SUGAR: 20G

CREAMY PEACH SMOOTHIE

GLUTEN FREE **QUICK & EASY** VEGETARIAN

SERVES 2 • PREP TIME: 10 MINUTES

Greek yogurt has a thick texture because the whey has been strained out of it. It also has a higher protein content than regular yogurt. Avoid sweetened yogurts because they can add a tremendous amount of sugar—up to 6 teaspoons per serving to your smoothie. If you are not restricting fat in your diet, a full-fat plain Greek yogurt is a nice alternative to 2-percent products.

2 cups 2% plain Greek yogurt

1 cup apple juice

1 frozen banana, sliced

1 cup chopped fresh peeled peaches

½ mango

2 tablespoons apple cider vinegar

1 tablespoon honey

Pinch of ground cinnamon

1. In a blender, combine the yogurt, apple juice, banana, peaches, mango, cider vinegar, honey, and cinnamon. Blend until smooth.

2. Pour into 2 tall glasses and serve.

 TIP To create a vegan smoothie, substitute a good-quality plain coconut yogurt or soy yogurt with no gelatin additives. If you use a vanilla-flavored yogurt, omit the honey.

PER SERVING CALORIES: 382; FAT: 5G; SATURATED FAT: 3G; PROTEIN: 25G; CARBS: 65G; SODIUM: 81MG; FIBER: 4G; SUGAR: 57G

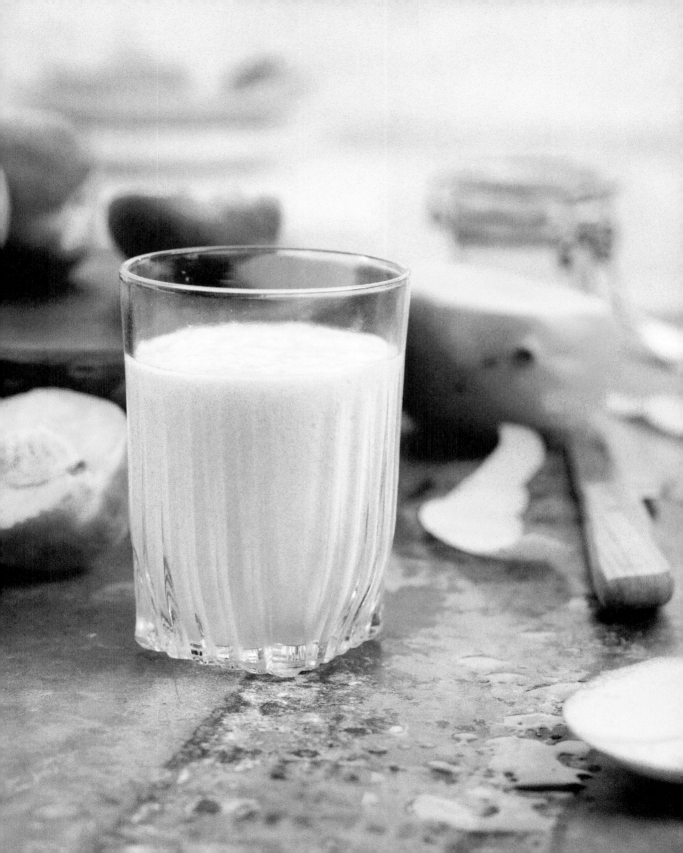

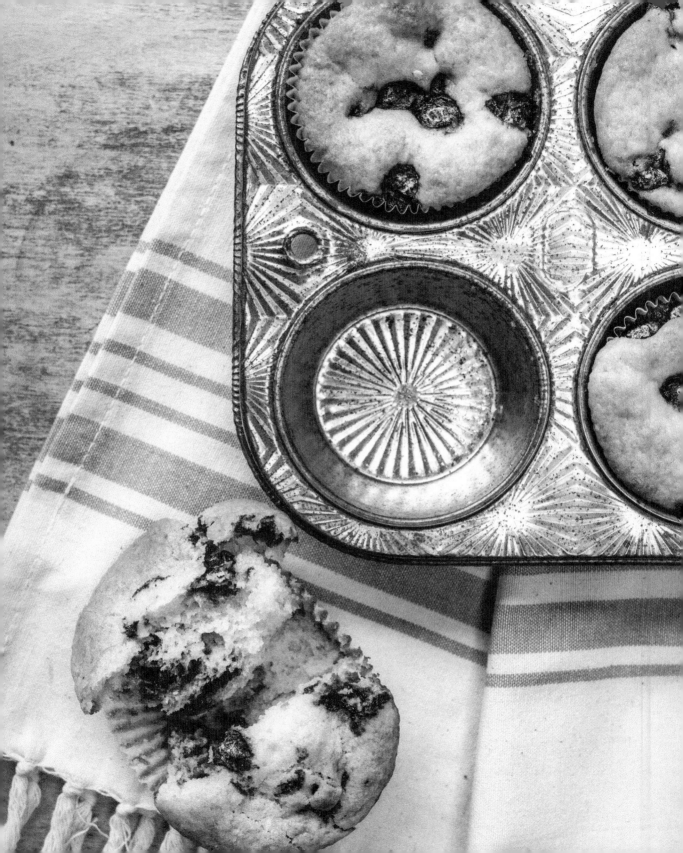

Chapter Seven

BREAKFAST

110   Blueberry Muffins

111   Cinnamon Apple Breakfast Cake

112   Irish Bannock

113   Bacon and Cheddar Breakfast Scones

114   Double Almond Muffins

115   Dark Chocolate Pancakes

116   Golden French Toast

118   Eggs Poached in Ratatouille

119   Creamy Scrambled Eggs

120   Flaky Biscuit and Egg Sandwiches

BLUEBERRY MUFFINS

VEGETARIAN

MAKES 12 MUFFINS • PREP TIME: 15 MINUTES • COOK TIME: 30 MINUTES

Blueberry muffins are a perfect choice to fill a pretty gift basket for a special friend. Tender, golden muffins studded with ripe, juicy blueberries look festive— and people will think you spent hours preparing them. You can use frozen berries, but thaw them first and don't stir the batter too much or it will turn purple.

2 cups whole milk

2 tablespoons apple cider vinegar

3½ cups all-purpose flour

¾ cup sugar

1 tablespoon baking soda

2 teaspoons ground cinnamon

Pinch of sea salt

½ cup melted coconut oil

2 tablespoons vanilla extract

2 cups fresh blueberries

1. Preheat the oven to 375°F. Line 12 muffin cups with paper liners.

2. In a small nonreactive bowl, whisk together the milk and cider vinegar. Set aside for 10 minutes.

3. In a large nonreactive bowl, stir together the flour, sugar, baking soda, cinnamon, and sea salt.

4. To the milk mixture, add the melted coconut oil and vanilla. Whisk until blended.

5. Add the milk mixture to the flour mixture and stir until just combined.

6. Gently fold the blueberries into the batter.

7. Spoon the batter into the muffin cups, filling three-fourths full.

8. Bake for 25 to 30 minutes, or until golden and a toothpick inserted in the center comes out clean.

9. Cool for 10 minutes before serving.

 TIP When you add a tablespoon of vinegar (or lemon juice) to a cup of milk and let it sit for 5 to 10 minutes, the milk will curdle, making a substitute for buttermilk, which contributes to the baking process and adds a bit of tangy flavor to the recipe.

PER SERVING (1 MUFFIN) CALORIES: 269; FAT: 11G; SATURATED FAT: 1G; PROTEIN: 5G; CARBS: 39G; SODIUM: 351MG; FIBER: 3G; SUGAR: 17G

CINNAMON APPLE BREAKFAST CAKE

VEGETARIAN

SERVES 8 • PREP TIME: 15 MINUTES • COOK TIME: 30 MINUTES

Cake for breakfast seems decadent, but this cake is healthy. Substitute almond flour for the all-purpose flour in the same quantities if you want a gluten-free cake, and use gluten-free baking powder and baking soda as well.

Butter, for the pan

1 cup all-purpose flour, plus additional for dusting

½ cup whole milk

2 tablespoons apple cider vinegar

4 tablespoons unsalted butter, at room temperature

¾ cup sugar

1 egg

1 teaspoon vanilla extract

1 teaspoon ground cinnamon

½ teaspoon baking powder

½ teaspoon baking soda

¼ teaspoon sea salt

1 cup chopped apple

1. Preheat the oven to 400°F. Lightly butter an 8-by-8-inch square baking pan and dust with flour.

2. In a small nonreactive bowl, stir together the milk and cider vinegar. Set aside for 10 minutes.

3. In a large nonreactive bowl, beat together the butter and sugar for about 3 minutes, until the mixture is fluffy, scraping down the sides of the bowl.

4. Add the egg and vanilla. Beat to combine.

5. In a medium bowl, stir together the flour, cinnamon, baking powder, baking soda, and sea salt.

6. Starting and ending with the flour mixture, alternately add the flour mixture and the milk mixture to the butter mixture in three additions. Beat after each addition to combine, and scrape down the sides of the bowl at least once.

7. Fold the apple into the batter. Pour the batter into the prepared pan.

8. Bake for 25 to 30 minutes, or until golden brown and a toothpick inserted in the center of the cake comes out clean.

9. Cool the cake in the pan for 10 minutes. Turn it out onto a wire rack to cool a bit more. Serve warm.

PER SERVING CALORIES: 207; FAT: 7G; SATURATED FAT: 4G;
PROTEIN: 3G; CARBS: 34G; SODIUM: 203MG; FIBER: 1G; SUGAR: 21G

IRISH BANNOCK

VEGETARIAN

SERVES 8 • PREP TIME: 20 MINUTES • COOK TIME: 45 MINUTES

Irish bannock has a long and interesting history as a flatbread, often made from oats and cooked on a griddle. Modern bannock is oven baked instead and is often used as a staple food for outdoor enthusiasts or eco-adventurers. This recipe is similar to Selkirk bannock, a Scottish variation, because of the raisins and currants added to the dough.

---

1 cup whole milk

2 tablespoons apple cider vinegar

2 cups all-purpose flour, plus more for dusting

¼ cup sugar

½ teaspoon baking soda

½ teaspoon baking powder

¼ teaspoon sea salt

¾ cup raisins

¼ cup currants

1. Preheat the oven to 375ºF. Line a baking sheet with parchment paper and spray it lightly with cooking oil.

2. In a small nonreactive bowl, stir together the milk and cider vinegar. Set aside for 10 minutes.

3. In a large nonreactive bowl, stir together the flour, sugar, baking soda, baking powder, and sea salt.

4. Stir the milk mixture into the flour mixture and, with your hands, mix the dough for about 5 minutes, or until it is soft and well combined. Add the raisins and currants. Mix with your hands to combine.

5. Lightly flour a clean work surface and turn the dough out onto the surface. Knead the dough for about 5 minutes, or until it is smooth and elastic. Form the dough into an 8-inch round and place it on the prepared pan. With a sharp knife, cut an X in the top of the dough.

6. Bake for about 45 minutes, or until golden and hollow sounding when tapped.

7. Cool for 10 minutes and serve warm.

 TIP Substituting almond milk or coconut milk in equal quantities for the whole milk can make this recipe suitable for vegans. The flavor might be altered slightly, but the texture should still be pleasing.

PER SERVING CALORIES: 199; FAT: 1G; SATURATED FAT: 1G; PROTEIN: 5G; CARBS: 43G; SODIUM: 168MG; FIBER: 2G; SUGAR: 16G

BACON AND CHEDDAR BREAKFAST SCONES

QUICK & EASY

MAKES 12 SCONES • PREP TIME: 15 MINUTES • COOK TIME: 15 MINUTES

If you want to intensify the bacon flavor in these scones, cook the bacon ahead of time and save the bacon fat in a small container in the freezer. When the bacon fat is solid, cut it into small pieces and use it instead of the butter in this recipe. Try a little chopped jalapeño, as well, for a spicy taste.

½ cup whole milk

2 tablespoons apple cider vinegar

2 cups all-purpose flour

1 tablespoon baking powder

½ teaspoon sea salt

½ teaspoon garlic powder

4 tablespoons cold butter, cut into small pieces

8 bacon slices, cooked and diced

1 cup shredded sharp Cheddar cheese

¼ cup maple syrup

1. Preheat the oven to 400°F. Line a baking sheet with parchment paper.

2. In a small nonreactive bowl, stir together the milk and cider vinegar. Set aside for 10 minutes.

3. In a food processor or blender, combine the flour, baking powder, sea salt, and garlic powder. Pulse for about 10 seconds to combine.

4. Add the cold butter pieces and pulse until the mixture resembles coarse crumbs.

5. Add the bacon and Cheddar cheese and pulse a couple of times to mix. Transfer the mixture to a large nonreactive bowl.

6. Add the milk mixture and maple syrup to the bowl. Stir until the batter pulls away from the sides of the bowl and holds together; do not overmix.

7. Scoop out ¼ cup of batter per scone and drop onto the prepared sheet. With your fingers, shape the scones into rough triangles.

8. Bake for about 15 minutes, or until golden.

9. Serve warm.

PER SERVING (1 SCONE) CALORIES: 237; FAT: 12G; SATURATED FAT: 6G; PROTEIN: 9G; CARBS: 22G; SODIUM: 477MG; FIBER: 1G; SUGAR: 5G

DOUBLE ALMOND MUFFINS

GLUTEN FREE **QUICK & EASY** VEGETARIAN

MAKES 12 MUFFINS • PREP TIME: 15 MINUTES • COOK TIME: 15 MINUTES

Honey adds sweetness and contributes to the tender crumb of these golden treats. Honey's flavor changes depending on the type of flowers bees have access to when collecting nectar. Alfalfa honey is delicate and flowery, while robust honey, such as buckwheat, is darker and full-bodied. Try several types to find your favorite.

---

3 cups almond flour

1 teaspoon baking soda

6 large eggs

3 tablespoons honey

1 tablespoon apple cider vinegar

1 teaspoon almond extract

1. Preheat the oven to 350°F. Line a 12-cup muffin tin with paper liners.

2. In a medium bowl, stir together the almond flour and baking soda.

3. In a large nonreactive bowl, whisk together the eggs, honey, cider vinegar, and almond extract until well blended.

4. Add the flour mixture to the egg mixture, and stir until just combined.

5. Scoop the batter into the prepared muffin cups, filling three-fourths full.

6. Bake for about 15 minutes, or until light golden brown.

7. Cool and serve.

 Almond flour comes in different consistencies, ranging from very fine to a moist meal. You can even make your own by blending blanched almonds in a food processor until they are ground. Try different types of almond flour for these muffins to create variations in taste and texture.

PER SERVING (1 MUFFIN) CALORIES: 92; FAT: 6G; SATURATED FAT: 1G; PROTEIN: 5G; CARBS: 6G; SODIUM: 142MG; FIBER: 1G; SUGAR: 6G

DARK CHOCOLATE PANCAKES

QUICK & EASY VEGETARIAN

SERVES 4 • PREP TIME: 10 MINUTES • COOK TIME: 20 MINUTES

Breakfast in bed for a loved one calls for a sumptuous dish. Top these with fresh strawberries, sliced banana, or a dollop of whipped cream. Refrigerate leftovers in a sealed plastic bag and pop them into the toaster to reheat.

---

2 cups whole milk

1 tablespoon apple cider vinegar

2 cups all-purpose flour

1 cup Dutch-processed cocoa powder

½ cup sugar

2 tablespoons baking powder

1 teaspoon ground cinnamon

Pinch of sea salt

¼ cup melted coconut oil

1 egg

1 tablespoon vanilla extract

Butter, for the skillet

1. In a medium nonreactive bowl, whisk together the milk and cider vinegar. Set aside for 10 minutes.

2. In a large nonreactive bowl, whisk together the flour, cocoa, sugar, baking powder, cinnamon, and sea salt until well mixed.

3. To the milk mixture, add the melted coconut oil, egg, and vanilla. Whisk until well blended. Add the milk mixture to the flour mixture, stirring until just combined.

4. Place a large nonstick skillet over medium heat and grease lightly with butter.

5. Spoon ¼ cup of pancake batter per pancake into the skillet, about 4 depending on the size of the skillet.

6. Cook for about 2 minutes, or until bubbles start to break on the surface. Flip and cook the other side for 1 to 2 minutes more, or until cooked through but still moist.

7. Transfer the pancakes to a warm plate to keep warm.

8. Repeat with the remaining batter. Serve warm.

 TIP Cocoa is a good source of iron, selenium, copper, magnesium, vitamin E, and several B vitamins. A tablespoon of cocoa powder also has about 1 gram of protein.

PER SERVING (2 PANCAKES) CALORIES: 542; FAT: 22G; SATURATED FAT: 5G; PROTEIN: 14G; CARBS: 83G; SODIUM: 135MG; FIBER: 9G; SUGAR: 32G

GOLDEN FRENCH TOAST

QUICK & EASY VEGETARIAN

SERVES 4 • PREP TIME: 20 MINUTES • COOK TIME: 10 MINUTES

Apple cider vinegar adds a delightful tang to the egg dip for the bread, which is also enhanced by vanilla and a hint of sweetness from the sugar. To make the dish ahead of time, dredge the bread in the egg mixture, shake off the excess liquid, place the bread on a baking sheet, and refrigerate the sheet, covered. Bake the French toast in a 350°F oven for 10 minutes, turning once, and serve.

¾ cup whole milk

¼ cup apple cider vinegar

3 eggs

2 tablespoons granulated sugar

1 teaspoon vanilla extract

8 thick bread slices

2 tablespoons butter, divided

Maple syrup, for serving

Fresh fruit (optional)

Confectioners' sugar (optional)

1. Preheat the oven to 200°F.

2. In a large nonreactive bowl, stir together the milk and cider vinegar. Set aside for 10 minutes.

3. To the milk mixture, whisk in the eggs, sugar, and vanilla.

4. Place a large skillet over medium-high heat and add 1 tablespoon of the butter.

5. Dip 4 bread slices into the egg mixture, turning them to soak.

6. Add the soaked bread to the skillet and cook for 2 minutes, turn, and continue cooking for 2 minutes more, or until the bread is golden brown and puffy. Transfer the French toast to a warm plate in the oven, and repeat with the remaining ingredients.

7. Serve warm topped with maple syrup, fresh fruit (if using), or a sprinkle of confectioners' sugar (if using).

PER SERVING CALORIES: 209; FAT: 12G; SATURATED FAT: 6G; PROTEIN: 8G; CARBS: 18G; SODIUM: 235MG; FIBER: 0G; SUGAR: 10G

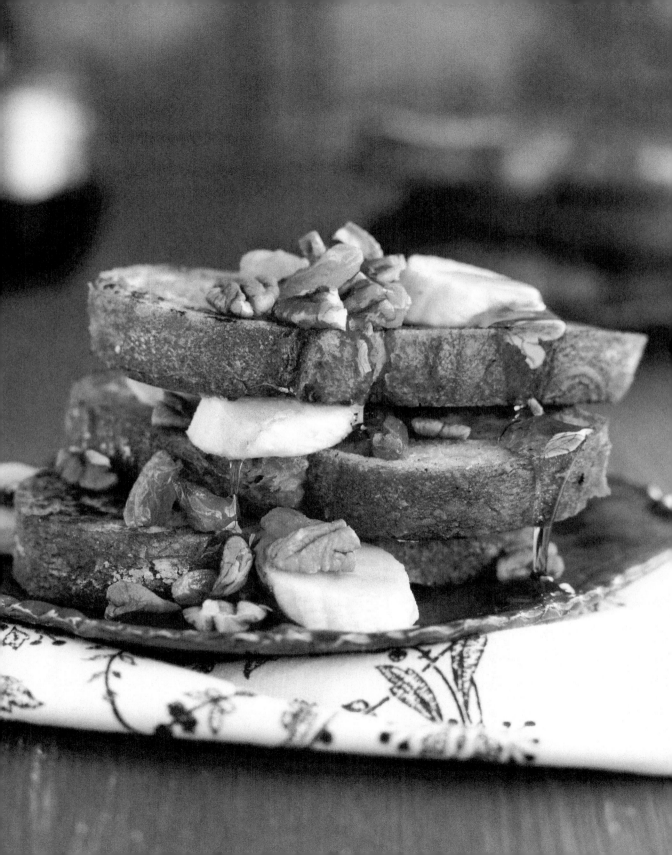

EGGS POACHED IN RATATOUILLE

GLUTEN FREE

SERVES 6 • PREP TIME: 15 MINUTES • COOK TIME: 45 MINUTES

French in origin, ratatouille is a simple dish whose name comes from the French word meaning to stir, touiller. *Ratatouille features a large dice of vegetables so each can still be recognized and the texture appreciated by the diners.*

2 teaspoons extra-virgin olive oil

1 large sweet onion, chopped

1 tablespoon minced garlic

1 small eggplant, peeled and diced

1 green zucchini, diced

1 yellow zucchini, diced

1 red bell pepper, diced

1 (28-ounce) can diced tomatoes

½ cup chicken broth

3 tablespoons apple cider vinegar

1 tablespoon chopped fresh basil

1 tablespoon chopped fresh oregano

Pinch red pepper flakes

6 eggs

1. In a large nonreactive skillet set over medium-high heat, heat the olive oil.

2. Add the onion and garlic. Sauté for about 3 minutes, or until the vegetables soften.

3. Stir in the eggplant, green zucchini, yellow zucchini, and bell pepper. Sauté for 5 minutes.

4. Stir in the tomatoes with their liquid, chicken broth, and cider vinegar. Bring to a boil. Reduce the heat to low and simmer for 30 minutes.

5. Stir in the basil, oregano, and red pepper flakes.

6. With the back of a large spoon, make 6 deep wells in the ratatouille. Crack 1 egg into each well. Cover the skillet and poach the eggs for 3 to 4 minutes, or until the whites are firm.

7. Serve one egg per person with a scoop of ratatouille.

 TIP The ratatouille can be made several days ahead and refrigerated until you are ready to serve. Simply reheat the ratatouille on the stove until it is piping hot before adding the eggs to poach.

PER SERVING CALORIES: 159; FAT: 7G; SATURATED FAT: 2G; PROTEIN: 10G; CARBS: 16G; SODIUM: 150MG; FIBER: 6G; SUGAR: 9G

CREAMY SCRAMBLED EGGS

GLUTEN FREE **QUICK & EASY** VEGETARIAN

SERVES 4 • PREP TIME: 15 MINUTES • COOK TIME: 5 MINUTES

Scrambling is a popular cooking method for eggs, but overstirring the raw mixture can create dry eggs. The trick is to swirl the pan when you pour the eggs into the skillet until cooked ridges form, then draw a spatula across the skillet to form moist, large egg curds. Move the cooked curds to the side of the skillet, off the heat, and continue moving the spatula until all the eggs are cooked.

¼ cup whole milk

2 tablespoons apple cider vinegar

8 eggs

1 tablespoon butter

Sea salt

Freshly ground black pepper

1 tablespoon chopped fresh chives

1. In a medium nonreactive bowl, stir together the milk and cider vinegar. Set aside for 10 minutes.

2. To the milk mixture, add the eggs and whisk to combine.

3. Place a large nonreactive skillet over medium-high heat and add the butter to melt.

4. Pour the eggs into the skillet. Cook for about 4 minutes, moving the eggs around with a spatula, until cooked through.

5. Season with sea salt and pepper.

6. Garnish with the chives and serve.

PER SERVING CALORIES: 179; FAT: 13G; SATURATED FAT: 5G;
PROTEIN: 13G; CARBS: 2G; SODIUM: 167MG; FIBER: 2G; SUGAR: 0G

FLAKY BISCUIT AND EGG SANDWICHES

VEGETARIAN

SERVES 8 • PREP TIME: 20 MINUTES • COOK TIME: 20 MINUTES

While baking is a science, biscuit making is also an art with regard to not overmixing the batter and achieving the perfect ratio of acid to fat. The folding technique in this recipe ensures that the biscuits are flaky. For extra layers, press the dough out again and refold it. Extra layers will also help keep it flaky if you plan to freeze the biscuit dough.

¾ cup whole milk

2 tablespoons apple cider vinegar

2 cups all-purpose flour, plus more for dusting

1 tablespoon baking powder

1 tablespoon sugar

1 teaspoon sea salt

½ cup (1 stick) cold butter, cut into pieces

2 tablespoons olive oil, divided

8 eggs

1. Preheat the oven to 450°F. Line a baking sheet with parchment paper.

2. In a small nonreactive bowl, stir together the milk and cider vinegar. Set aside for 10 minutes.

3. In a large nonreactive bowl, whisk together the flour, baking powder, sugar, and sea salt.

4. Add the butter to the flour mixture. Using two knives or a pastry blender, cut the butter into the dry ingredients until it resembles pea-size chunks.

5. Add the milk mixture, stirring until the batter is just combined.

6. Lightly flour a clean work surface and turn the dough out onto it.

7. Pat the dough into a rectangle. Fold the long sides in toward the middle, like folding a letter. Pat the dough again to form a 6 by 9-inch rectangle about 1 inch thick.

8. With a 2-inch biscuit cutter, make 8 biscuits and place them on the prepared sheet. Gather together the scraps of dough and cut out more biscuits.

9. Bake for about 10 minutes, or until golden brown. Set aside to cool on a rack while you cook the eggs.

10. Line a large plate with paper towels. Place a large skillet over medium-high heat and add 1 tablespoon of the olive oil.

11. Crack 4 eggs into the hot skillet. Fry for about 4 minutes, or until the whites set and the yolks are firm but still runny. Transfer to a paper towel–lined plate. Repeat with the remaining 1 tablespoon olive oil and 4 eggs.

12. Cut the biscuits in half. Top each bottom half with 1 egg. Top with the biscuit top. Serve hot.

TIP Top the egg sandwiches with sliced tomato, bacon, or cheese. You can halve this recipe if you do not need 8 biscuit sandwiches, but the leftover biscuits are fabulous as a snack with a little butter and jam.

PER SERVING CALORIES: 339; FAT: 21G; SATURATED FAT: 9G; PROTEIN: 10G; CARBS: 28G; SODIUM: 454MG; FIBER: 1G; SUGAR: 3G

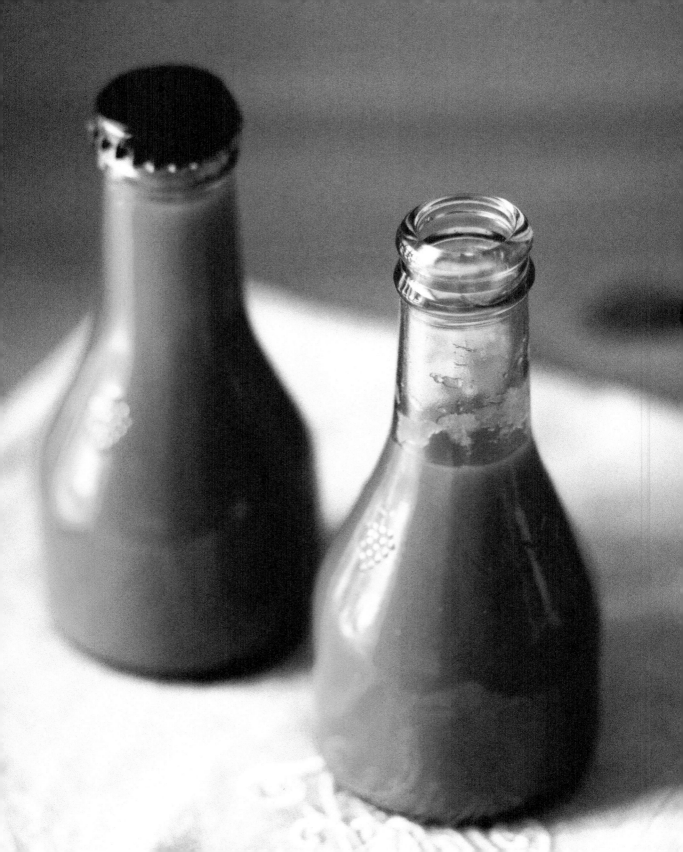

Chapter Eight

CONDIMENTS & SIDES

124	Tomato Ketchup
125	Sweet and Spicy Barbecue Sauce
126	Berry Vinaigrette
128	Sun-Dried Tomato Vinaigrette
129	Green Goddess Dressing
130	Herb-Flower Vinegar
131	Roasted Maple Celeriac
133	Garlic Dill Pickles
134	Creamy Mashed Potatoes
135	Bavarian Braised Red Cabbage

TOMATO KETCHUP

GLUTEN FREE **PALEO FRIENDLY** QUICK & EASY **VEGAN** VEGETARIAN

MAKES 3 CUPS • PREP TIME: 10 MINUTES

Prepared ketchup is a high-sodium food—a fact that is often overlooked by people watching their diets. One-quarter cup of ketchup can contain over 650 mg of sodium, which is more than five times the amount found in this tasty homemade version. Do not substitute other spices for the cloves and allspice in this recipe, because they create the distinctive "ketchup" flavor.

---

3 (6-ounce) cans tomato paste

6 tablespoons apple cider vinegar

6 tablespoons honey

½ teaspoon ground cloves

½ teaspoon sea salt

¼ teaspoon ground allspice

Water, for thinning

1. In a large nonreactive bowl, whisk together the tomato paste, cider vinegar, honey, cloves, sea salt, and allspice until very smooth.

2. Add enough water to achieve the desired consistency.

3. Refrigerate the ketchup in a sealed container for up to 2 weeks.

PER SERVING (¼ CUP) CALORIES: 69; FAT: 0G; SATURATED FAT: 0G; PROTEIN: 2G; CARBS: 17G; SODIUM: 121MG; FIBER: 2G; SUGAR: 14G

SWEET AND SPICY BARBECUE SAUCE

GLUTEN FREE **PALEO FRIENDLY** QUICK & EASY **VEGAN** VEGETARIAN

MAKES 1½ CUPS • PREP TIME: 5 MINUTES • COOK TIME: 5 MINUTES

Great barbecue sauce can be brushed on many different meats and poultry, as well as poured on hamburgers and stirred into baked beans. Barbecue sauce needs to be thin enough so it doesn't mask the natural flavor of your protein and thick enough not to run off. Make a double batch in the summer when barbecuing is a popular cooking choice.

---

1 (6-ounce) can tomato paste

¼ cup apple cider vinegar

¼ cup water

2 tablespoons molasses

2 tablespoons honey

1 tablespoon extra-virgin olive oil

1 tablespoon onion powder

2 teaspoons garlic powder

1 teaspoon chili powder

¼ teaspoon cayenne pepper

¼ teaspoon sea salt

1. In a small nonreactive saucepan, whisk together the tomato paste, cider vinegar, water, molasses, honey, olive oil, onion powder, garlic powder, chili powder, cayenne pepper, and sea salt.

2. Place the saucepan over medium heat and bring the sauce to a boil. Boil for about 5 minutes, stirring. Remove from the heat and let cool.

3. Refrigerate the sauce in a sealed glass container for up to 2 weeks.

 TIP Molasses comes in several different types—light, dark, and blackstrap molasses in most stores—and the final taste of this sauce depends on which type you use. Blackstrap molasses will impart the smokiest taste, but dark molasses is appropriate, as well.

PER SERVING (¼ CUP) CALORIES: 95; FAT: 3G; SATURATED FAT: 0G;
PROTEIN: 2G; CARBS: 18G; SODIUM: 115MG; FIBER: 2G; SUGAR: 14G

BERRY VINAIGRETTE

GLUTEN FREE **PALEO FRIENDLY QUICK & EASY VEGAN** VEGETARIAN

MAKES 2 CUPS • PREP TIME: 10 MINUTES

Tiny deep-green flecks of basil look gorgeous suspended in this pink-hued vinaigrette. Basil also provides vitamin K, manganese, and copper along with disease-fighting flavonoids. This fragrant herb is a powerful antibacterial, which means the essential oils in the leaves inhibit bacterial growth in your finished dressing.

½ cup apple cider vinegar

¼ cup fresh strawberries

¼ cup fresh raspberries

1 tablespoon honey

¼ teaspoon chopped fresh basil

Pinch of sea salt

¾ cup extra-virgin olive oil

1. In a blender, combine the cider vinegar, strawberries, raspberries, honey, basil, and sea salt. Pulse for about 20 seconds, or until blended.

2. Pour in the olive oil. Pulse for about 15 seconds, or until emulsified.

3. Refrigerate in a sealed container for up to 1 week.

4. Shake before using.

 If you do not live in an area with a bounty of fresh berries or you want to make this vinaigrette when these fruits are out of season, frozen berries will work. Thaw them first before blending into the other ingredients.

PER SERVING (2 TABLESPOONS) CALORIES: 88; FAT: 10G; SATURATED FAT: 1G; PROTEIN: 0G; CARBS: 2G; SODIUM: 16MG; FIBER: 0G; SUGAR: 1G

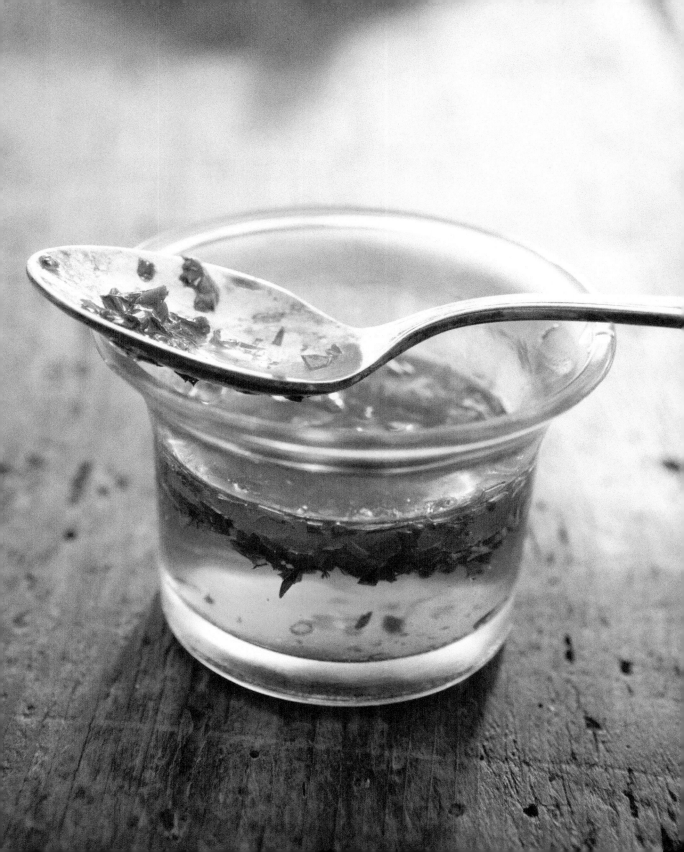

SUN-DRIED TOMATO VINAIGRETTE

GLUTEN FREE **PALEO FRIENDLY** QUICK & EASY **VEGAN** VEGETARIAN

MAKES 2 CUPS • PREP TIME: 10 MINUTES

Drying tomatoes in the sun (or in an oven) is an effective method to preserve delicate tomatoes without losing their health benefits. You will find that sun-dried tomatoes have a sweeter taste than fresh ones and a pleasing chewy texture. Sun-dried tomatoes are an excellent source of potassium, iron, manganese, magnesium, copper, and phosphorus.

12 oil-packed sun-dried tomatoes, chopped

½ cup cherry tomatoes, halved

¼ cup apple cider vinegar

1 teaspoon minced garlic

1 tablespoon chopped fresh basil

1 teaspoon chopped fresh oregano

1 cup extra-virgin olive oil

Sea salt

Freshly ground black pepper

1. In a blender, combine the sun-dried tomatoes, cherry tomatoes, cider vinegar, garlic, basil, and oregano. Pulse for about 30 seconds, or until finely chopped.

2. Pour in the olive oil. Pulse for about 1 minute, or until the vinaigrette is emulsified and smooth.

3. Season the vinaigrette with sea salt and pepper and pulse again to combine.

4. Refrigerate in a sealed container for up to 2 weeks.

5. Shake before using.

PER SERVING (2 TABLESPOONS) CALORIES: 115; FAT: 13G; SATURATED FAT: 2G; PROTEIN: 0G; CARBS: 1G; SODIUM: 7MG; FIBER: 0G; SUGAR: 0G

GREEN GODDESS DRESSING

GLUTEN FREE **PALEO FRIENDLY** QUICK & EASY **VEGAN** VEGETARIAN

MAKES 2 CUPS • PREP TIME: 10 MINUTES

The first green goddess dressing was named to recognize English actor George Arliss and a play he starred in called The Green Goddess *in San Francisco in the 1920s. The Palace Hotel chef honored the actor and the play, which was made into a movie considered the earliest "talkie." Green goddess dressing traditionally includes anchovies, but this version is still delicious without them.*

1 medium avocado, peeled and pitted

1 scallion, both white and green parts, chopped

1 cup fresh basil

¼ cup extra-virgin olive oil

¼ cup water, plus more as needed

¼ cup chopped fresh parsley

Juice of 1 large lemon

2 tablespoons apple cider vinegar

1 teaspoon honey

½ teaspoon minced garlic

½ teaspoon sea salt

1. In a food processor, combine the avocado, scallion, basil, olive oil, water, and parsley. Pulse until blended.

2. Add the lemon juice, cider vinegar, honey, garlic, and sea salt. Process until well blended.

3. If the dressing is too thick, add more water a little bit at a time.

4. Refrigerate in a sealed container for up to 2 weeks.

PER SERVING (2 TABLESPOONS) CALORIES: 56; FAT: 6G; SATURATED FAT: 1G; PROTEIN: 0G; CARBS: 2G; SODIUM: 60MG; FIBER: 1G; SUGAR: 0G

HERB-FLOWER VINEGAR

GLUTEN FREE **PALEO FRIENDLY VEGAN** VEGETARIAN

MAKES 4 CUPS • PREP TIME: 15 MINUTES, PLUS 2 WEEKS, INFUSION TIME • COOK TIME: 2 MINUTES

Adding herbs to your culinary creations can introduce new flavors and provide untold health benefits to your family. Herbal vinegars can be delicious in sauces, salads, and gravies. They also are very attractive displayed on a counter, useful as a housewarming gift, or as a hostess gift.

1¼ cups chopped organic herb flowers, such as lavender, chive flowers, rose petals, thyme, sweet violets, or nasturtiums, picked through, stems and damaged parts removed

4 cups apple cider vinegar, divided

Herb flower sprigs, for decorating

1. In a large nonreactive bowl, add the flowers and lightly crush selected ones with the back of a spoon.

2. Place a small nonreactive saucepan over medium heat. Add 2 cups of the cider vinegar. Heat the vinegar for about 2 minutes, or until warm. Pour over the crushed flowers.

3. With a spoon, press the flowers into the vinegar to release their flavor. Cool the mixture.

4. Stir the remaining 2 cups cider vinegar into the bowl to combine.

5. Transfer the floral vinegar into clean sealable jars. Seal with acid-proof lids.

6. Place the sealed jars in a sunny area for 2 weeks, shaking the jars every day.

7. If you want a stronger floral flavor, strain the vinegar and discard the flowers. Repeat the process with fresh flowers.

8. Strain the finished infused vinegar through fine cheesecloth and pour into decorative bottles. Place a fresh herb flower sprig into the finished product and seal.

9. Store in a cool, dark place for up to 1 month.

 TIP Only use organic blossoms in this recipe to avoid pesticide contamination. These flowers can be found in many specialty produce stores or you can grow your own to be sure of their origin.

PER SERVING (2 TABLESPOONS) CALORIES: 6G; FAT: 0G; SATURATED FAT: 0G; PROTEIN: 0G; CARBS: 0G; SODIUM: 22G; FIBER: 0G; SUGAR: 0G

ROASTED MAPLE CELERIAC

GLUTEN FREE **PALEO FRIENDLY** **VEGAN** VEGETARIAN

SERVES 4 • PREP TIME: 15 MINUTES • COOK TIME: 20 MINUTES

If you're unfamiliar with celeriac (celery root), you might be surprised when you first see it. This flavorful vegetable looks like a dirty ball of gnarled roots, and a little scaly depending on its age. Once you wash off the dirt and cut off the strange skin, you will be delighted with the fresh, almost parsley-like scent of its creamy root flesh.

---

2 celeriac roots, peeled and diced into 1-inch pieces

2 teaspoons extra-virgin olive oil

Pinch of sea salt

2 tablespoons apple cider vinegar

2 tablespoons maple syrup

¼ teaspoon ground ginger

Freshly ground black pepper

1. Preheat the oven to 400°F. Line a baking sheet with parchment paper.

2. In a large bowl, toss together the celeriac, olive oil, and sea salt.

3. Spread the vegetable on the prepared sheet. Roast for about 20 minutes, or until very tender and lightly caramelized.

4. Transfer the celeriac to a large nonreactive bowl. Add the cider vinegar, maple syrup, and ginger. With a potato masher, mash the ingredients to the desired texture.

5. Season with pepper and serve warm.

TIP Celeriac is an often underutilized root vegetable that is low in calories; a half cup has less than 20 calories. Celeriac is a good source of fiber, vitamin C, iron, potassium, and phosphorus. This tasty vegetable is a smart choice for any weight-loss diet.

PER SERVING CALORIES: 56; FAT: 2G; SATURATED FAT: 0G; PROTEIN: 0G; CARBS: 9G; SODIUM: 117MG; FIBER: 1G; SUGAR: 7G

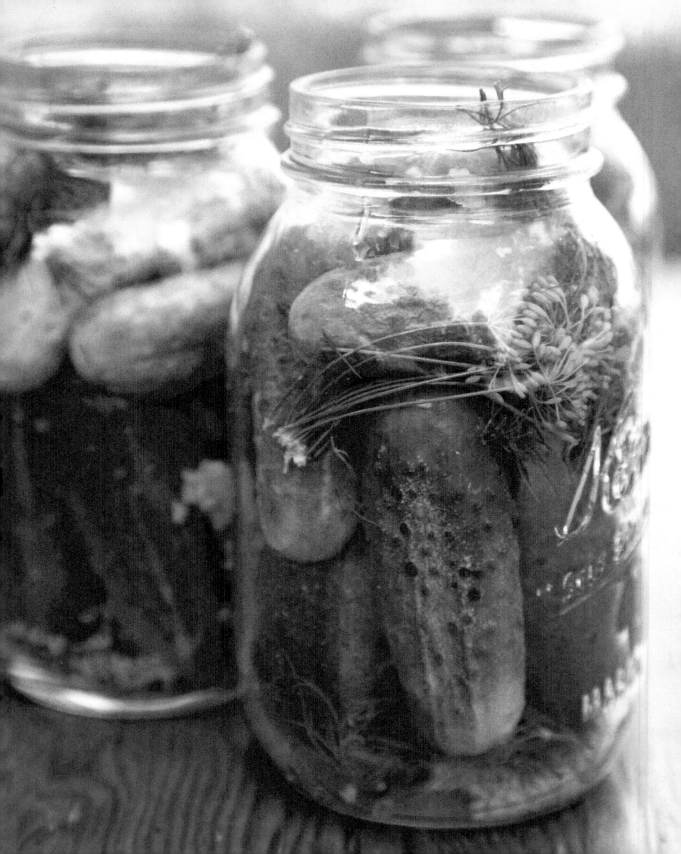

GARLIC DILL PICKLES

GLUTEN FREE **PALEO FRIENDLY VEGAN** VEGETARIAN

MAKES 1 QUART • PREP TIME: 30 MINUTES, PLUS 1 WEEK PICKLING TIME • COOK TIME: 20 MINUTES

One of the oldest preservation methods for vegetables, pickling ensured that people had enough food stores to survive the winter. This recipe can be doubled, tripled, and even quadrupled if you have a large amount of pickling cucumbers. These small, thin-skinned vegetables are not just immature salad cucumbers, but rather varieties that are crisper, more flavorful, and naturally tiny.

¾ cup filtered water, plus more for sterilizing

¾ cup apple cider vinegar

1 tablespoon pickling salt

4 garlic cloves

2 teaspoons dill seed

2 dill sprigs

1 teaspoon black peppercorns

1½ pounds pickling cucumbers, thoroughly washed and any bruised vegetables discarded

1. Place a 1-quart glass jar, or two 1-pint jars, in a large pot. Cover the jar(s) with filtered water by about 2 inches. Place the pot over high heat and bring to a boil.

2. Boil for 15 minutes. Turn off the heat. With tongs, remove the jars and set aside to cool. Add the canning lid(s) to the hot water and leave there until needed.

3. In a medium nonreactive saucepan set over high heat, stir together the cider vinegar, ¾ cup of filtered water, and pickling salt. Bring to a boil. Remove from the heat.

4. Place the garlic, dill seed, dill sprigs, and peppercorns in the 1-quart jar, or evenly divide between the two 1-pint jars.

5. Pack the cucumbers in the jar(s) as tightly as possible.

6. Pour the hot vinegar brine into the jar(s), leaving about ¼ inch of headspace.

7. Gently tap the jar(s) on the counter to remove any air bubbles.

8. Carefully wipe the jar rims clean. Apply the lids and bands until they are just secure; don't screw them on too tightly.

9. Cool the jars completely and then refrigerate.

10. Let the pickles sit for at least 1 week before eating and keep them refrigerated. They will keep in the refrigerator for up to 1 month.

PER SERVING (2 PICKLES) CALORIES: 22; FAT: 0G; SATURATED FAT: 0G; PROTEIN: 2G; CARBS: 4G; SODIUM: 723MG; FIBER: 1G; SUGAR: 2G

CREAMY MASHED POTATOES

GLUTEN FREE **QUICK & EASY** VEGETARIAN

SERVES 4 • PREP TIME: 10 MINUTES • COOK TIME: 20 MINUTES

Certain potato varieties are better than others for mashing. To avoid a lumpy, gooey texture, you need mashing potatoes with a high starch content. Good mashing potatoes fall apart when mashed, whip up fluffy, and readily absorb liquid, such as the apple cider–spiked milk in this recipe. Russets potatoes are excellent high-starch choices.

2 pounds russet potatoes, peeled and cut into chunks

½ cup whole milk

1 tablespoon apple cider vinegar

Sea salt

Freshly ground black pepper

1. In a large nonreactive saucepan, combine the potatoes and enough cold water to cover by 2 inches. Add a pinch of sea salt. Bring the water to a boil over high heat. Reduce the heat to a simmer. Cook for 15 to 20 minutes, or until the potatoes are fork-tender.

2. In small nonreactive bowl, stir together the milk and cider vinegar. Set aside for 10 minutes.

3. Drain the potatoes well. Return them to the pot. Add the milk mixture and mash until smooth and fluffy.

4. Season with sea salt and pepper before serving hot.

PER SERVING CALORIES: 176; FAT: 1G; SATURATED FAT: 1G; PROTEIN: 5G; CARBS: 37G; SODIUM: 96MG; FIBER: 5G; SUGAR: 4G

BAVARIAN BRAISED RED CABBAGE

GLUTEN FREE **VEGETARIAN**

SERVES 4 • PREP TIME: 20 MINUTES • COOK TIME: 1 HOUR

When braised, red cabbage becomes a rich, dark magenta and adds stunning color as a side dish for any meal. Cabbage can lower cholesterol levels and help fight several types of cancer, such as colon, bladder, and prostate cancer. This pretty, red cruciferous vegetable has more disease-busting antioxidants than its green counterparts and is a fantastic source of vitamins C and K.

1 red cabbage, cored and finely shredded

1 large sweet onion, sliced thin

1 cup apple cider vinegar

½ cup vegetable broth

¼ cup sugar

1 teaspoon sea salt

2 tablespoons butter

1. In a large nonreactive saucepan set over medium-high heat, add the red cabbage, onion, cider vinegar, vegetable broth, sugar, and sea salt and stir. Bring to a boil.

2. Reduce the heat to low. Simmer for about 1 hour, or until the vegetables are very tender and the liquid is almost evaporated, stirring frequently.

3. Stir in the butter and serve hot.

 If you want to make a large batch or don't have an hour to watch the pot, use a slow cooker. Mix all the ingredients together in the slow cooker. Cover and cook on low for 6 to 8 hours.

PER SERVING CALORIES: 172; FAT: 6G; SATURATED FAT: 4G; PROTEIN: 3G; CARBS: 27G; SODIUM: 567MG; FIBER: 5G; SUGAR: 20G

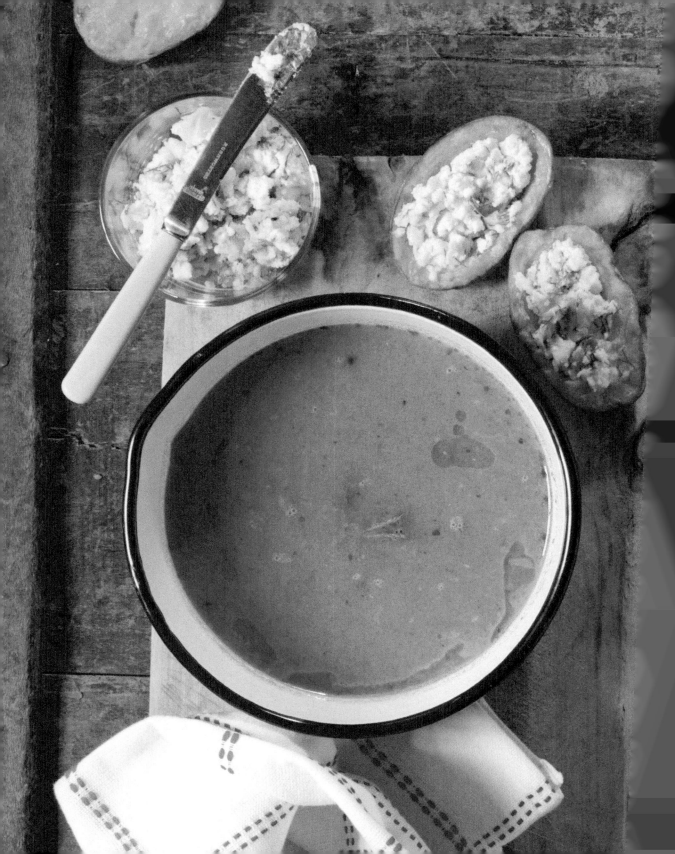

Chapter Nine

SOUPS & SALADS

138   Homemade Beef Stock

139   Homemade Chicken Stock

140   Hot and Sour Soup

141   Chicken-Broccoli Soup

142   Curried Root Vegetable Soup

144   Roasted Tomato Soup

145   Oktoberfest Stew

146   Mustard Chicken Salad

147   Spiced Carrot Salad

149   Greek Couscous Salad

150   Grilled Vegetable Pasta Salad

151   Potato Salad with Hot Bacon Dressing

152   Fennel-Jicama Salad

154   Asian Asparagus Salad

155   Watermelon-Tomato Salad

HOMEMADE BEEF STOCK

GLUTEN FREE **PALEO FRIENDLY**

MAKES 10 TO 12 CUPS • PREP TIME: 20 MINUTES • COOK TIME: 18 HOURS, 45 MINUTES

Beef bone broth is fast becoming a culinary sensation with those who take their health seriously. Slow cooking roasted bones with vegetables for added flavor and apple cider vinegar to leach minerals from the bones creates a deliciously nourishing food that speeds healing and provides easily digestible nutrients. This elixir can prevent disease and reduce symptoms of an existing condition.

3 pounds beef bones, ribs, beef marrow, knuckles, and any other bones

2 carrots, chopped into 1-inch pieces

2 celery stalks, cut into large chunks

1 onion, peeled and quartered

5 garlic cloves, lightly crushed

10 black peppercorns

3 dried bay leaves

Water, for cooking

¼ cup apple cider vinegar

1. Preheat the oven to 350°F.

2. Add the beef bones to a roasting pan. Roast for 45 minutes.

3. With tongs, transfer the bones to a large nonreactive stockpot. Add the carrots, celery, onion, garlic, peppercorns, and bay leaves. Add enough water to cover the bones by about 4 inches. Stir in the cider vinegar.

4. Place the pot over high heat and bring to a boil. Reduce the heat to low so the stock simmers gently, and cover the pot. Check the stock every hour, skimming off any foam that forms on top. Simmer the stock for 18 hours.

5. Remove the pot from the heat. Cool the stock for 45 minutes. With tongs, remove the larger bones.

6. Using a fine sieve, strain the stock into a large nonreactive bowl. Discard the leftover vegetables and bones. Let the broth cool a bit.

7. Transfer the broth to clean jars and let cool. Seal the jars.

8. Refrigerate for up to 5 days, or keep in the freezer for up to 2 months.

 TIP Beef bones are readily available in most grocery stores or local butchers. You can often find them packaged in the meat department. If you don't, ask the butcher for assistance or to save the bones for you.

PER SERVING CALORIES: 66; FAT: 3G; SATURATED FAT: 1 G; PROTEIN: 4G; CARBS: 1G; SODIUM: 287MG; FIBER: 0G; SUGAR: 1G

HOMEMADE CHICKEN STOCK

GLUTEN FREE **PALEO FRIENDLY**

MAKES 8 TO 10 CUPS • PREP TIME: 15 MINUTES • COOK TIME: 18 HOURS, 45 MINUTES

The belief that homemade chicken soup can cure the common cold, and other ailments, might have a solid basis in science. Many think the vegetables and meat in the soup help heal the body. But if you removed all the solids from your favorite chicken soup recipe, leaving just this tasty bone broth, you still might feel better. Chicken contains cysteine, a natural amino acid that can thin congesting mucus in the lungs, making it easier to breathe. When you have roast chicken for dinner, seal the meatless carcass in a resealable plastic bag and store in the freezer (up to 2 months) until you have two carcasses and can make this stock.

2 chicken carcasses

3 celery stalks with leaves, quartered

2 carrots, chopped into 2-inch pieces

1 large sweet onion, peeled and quartered

4 garlic cloves, lightly crushed

10 black peppercorns

4 fresh thyme sprigs

3 dried bay leaves

Water, for cooking

3 tablespoons apple cider vinegar

1. Preheat the oven to 350°F.

2. Add the chicken carcasses to a deep roasting pan. Roast for 45 minutes.

3. Transfer the roasted carcasses to a large nonreactive stockpot. Add the celery, carrots, onion, garlic, peppercorns, thyme, and bay leaves. Add enough water to cover the bones and vegetables by about 4 inches. Stir in the cider vinegar.

4. Place the pot on high heat and bring to a boil. Reduce the heat to low. Check the stock every hour, skimming off any foam that forms on top. Simmer the stock for 18 hours.

5. Remove the pot from the heat. Cool the stock for 45 minutes. With tongs, remove any large bones.

6. Using a fine sieve, strain the stock into a large nonreactive bowl. Discard any leftover bones and vegetables.

7. Transfer the stock to clean jars and cool completely. Seal the jars.

8. Refrigerate for up to 5 days, or store in the freezer for up to 2 months.

PER SERVING CALORIES: 54; FAT: 3G; SATURATED FAT: 1G;
PROTEIN: 6G; CARBS: 8G; SODIUM: 213MG; FIBER: 0G; SUGAR: 0G

HOT AND SOUR SOUP

GLUTEN FREE **QUICK & EASY**

MAKES 4 SERVINGS • PREP TIME: 15 MINUTES • COOK TIME: 15 MINUTES

The final splash of vinegar to this soup's broth is crucial for creating the signature sour taste—use either the recommended amount or a little more, depending on your palate. Include extra-firm tofu if you want more protein and bulk in the soup. The cornstarch mixed with the egg helps hold the egg together better and thickens the soup.

4 teaspoons apple cider vinegar

1 tablespoon low-sodium soy sauce

1 teaspoon sugar

½ teaspoon freshly ground black pepper

Pinch of red pepper flakes

1 teaspoon sesame oil

1 cup sliced mushrooms

2 teaspoons grated fresh peeled ginger

1 cup chopped cooked chicken breast

8 cups low-sodium chicken broth

2 eggs, beaten

1 teaspoon cornstarch

4 medium bok choy, washed and julienned

1 red bell pepper, trimmed, seeded, and julienned

1 scallion, finely chopped

1. In a small nonreactive bowl, stir together the cider vinegar, soy sauce, sugar, black pepper, and red pepper flakes. Set aside.

2. Place a large nonreactive soup pot over medium-high heat. Add the sesame oil.

3. Add the mushrooms and ginger. Sauté for about 3 minutes, or until translucent.

4. Add the chicken. Sauté for 2 minutes.

5. Pour in the chicken broth and the reserved vinegar mixture. Bring the soup to a boil.

6. In a small bowl, whisk together the eggs and cornstarch. In a thin stream, gently stir the eggs into the soup.

7. Reduce the heat to low. Add the bok choy and bell pepper. Simmer for about 5 minutes. Remove from the heat.

8. Garnish with the scallion and serve immediately.

 TIP After adding the eggs, stir the soup gently to avoid breaking up the cooked egg strands. The noodle-like strands of egg swirling in the flavorful broth are one of the best elements of hot and sour soup.

PER SERVING CALORIES: 251; FAT: 7G; SATURATED FAT: 1G; PROTEIN: 31G; CARBS: 23G; SODIUM: 971MG; FIBER: 10G; SUGAR: 13G

CHICKEN-BROCCOLI SOUP

GLUTEN FREE **PALEO FRIENDLY**

SERVES 6 • PREP TIME: 20 MINUTES • COOK TIME: 35 MINUTES

Leftover chicken or turkey can be put to tasty use in a simple vegetable soup. Any combination of vegetables can be used, as well as thin egg noodles or alphabet pasta, depending on what's in your cupboard or refrigerator and how many people you want to feed. Broccoli slaw is a good inclusion in this soup because the flavor of the shredded stalks is strong and it holds texture in a simmering soup.

1 tablespoon extra-virgin olive oil

1 small sweet onion, chopped

2 teaspoons minced garlic

3 celery stalks with leaves, chopped

2 carrots, diced

2 cups chopped cooked chicken

8 cups chicken broth

3 tablespoons apple cider vinegar

2 cups broccoli slaw

2 tablespoons chopped fresh thyme

2 tablespoons chopped fresh parsley

Sea salt

Freshly ground black pepper

1. Place a large nonreactive stockpot over medium-high heat and add the olive oil.

2. Add the onion and garlic. Sauté for about 3 minutes, or until translucent.

3. Add the celery and carrots. Sauté for 2 minutes.

4. Stir in the chicken, chicken broth, and cider vinegar. Bring to a boil. Reduce the heat to low and simmer for 20 minutes.

5. Stir in the broccoli slaw, thyme, and parsley. Simmer the soup for 10 minutes more.

6. Season with sea salt and pepper and serve hot.

 Broccoli slaw is available in large or small packages in the produce section of most grocery stores, usually next to the pre-packaged coleslaw. You can shred fresh broccoli at home, but use only the stalks for slaw, because the florets will get soggy and overcooked in this soup.

PER SERVING CALORIES: 127; FAT: 4G; SATURATED FAT: 1G; PROTEIN: 16G; CARBS: 6G; SODIUM: 455MG; FIBER: 2G; SUGAR: 2G

CURRIED ROOT VEGETABLE SOUP

GLUTEN FREE VEGETARIAN

SERVES 6 • PREP TIME: 30 MINUTES • COOK TIME: 35 MINUTES

Make this robust dish even heartier by thickening it at the end with cornstarch, and serve smaller amounts over rice or noodles. If a vegan dish is required, simply swap the butter for olive oil and omit the cream finish.

2 tablespoons butter

½ sweet onion, chopped

1 leek, white and pale green parts only, thoroughly washed and chopped

1 celery stalk, chopped

1 teaspoon minced garlic

1 teaspoon grated fresh peeled ginger

½ pound carrots, peeled and chopped

½ pound parsnips, peeled and chopped

1 apple, peeled, cored, and chopped

1 tablespoon curry powder

¼ teaspoon cayenne pepper

5 cups vegetable broth

½ cup heavy (whipping) cream

2 tablespoons apple cider vinegar

Sea salt

Freshly ground black pepper

2 tablespoons chopped fresh cilantro

4 teaspoons chopped shelled pumpkin seeds (pepitas)

1. Place a large nonreactive saucepan over medium-high heat and melt the butter.

2. Add the onion, leek, celery, garlic, and ginger. Sauté for about 5 minutes, or until softened. Add the carrots, parsnips, apple, curry powder, and cayenne pepper. Sauté for 3 minutes.

3. Stir in the vegetable broth. Bring to a boil. Reduce the heat to low, and simmer for about 25 minutes, stirring occasionally, or until the vegetables are very tender. Remove from the heat.

4. Stir in the heavy cream. Stir in the cider vinegar.

5. In a food processor or blender, purée the soup in batches until very smooth.

6. Transfer the soup to a saucepan and reheat over low heat. Season with sea salt and pepper. Top with cilantro and pepitas before serving hot.

 TIP When puréeing hot soup, use small batches. Remove the plug in the lid, cover the lid with a doubled clean cloth, and hold the lid down. The lid opening will allow the steam to escape, so the soup won't overflow.

PER SERVING CALORIES: 157; FAT: 8G; SATURATED FAT: 5G;
PROTEIN: 3G; CARBS: 20G; SODIUM: 109MG; FIBER: 5G; SUGAR: 9G

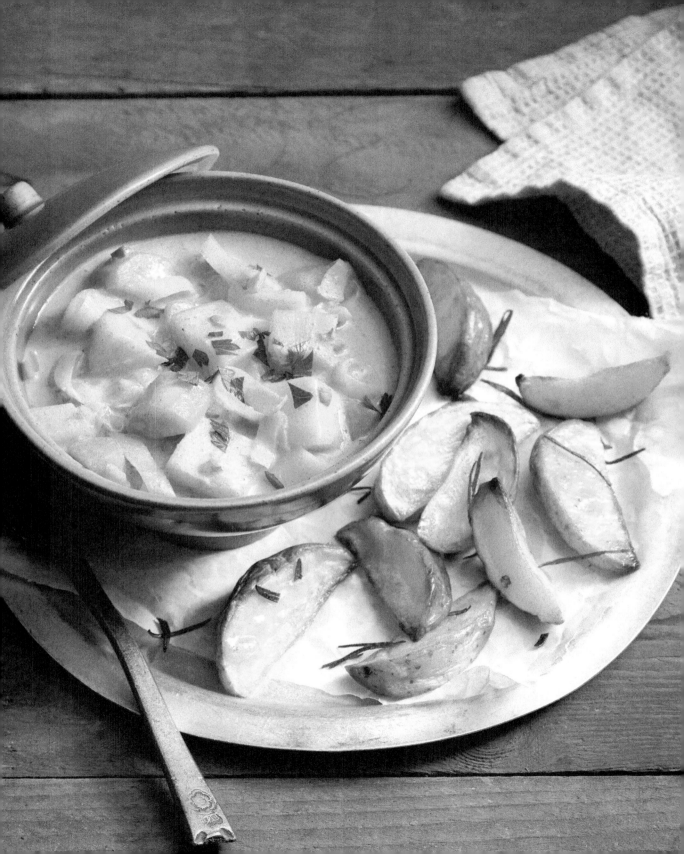

ROASTED TOMATO SOUP

GLUTEN FREE

SERVES 4 • PREP TIME: 15 MINUTES • COOK TIME: 40 TO 45 MINUTES

Leftovers are unlikely when you purée a batch of this soup, because the sweet, smoky taste is almost addictive. If you happen to end up with a few extra cups, heat it and toss it, along with a couple tablespoons of Parmesan cheese, with some cooked pasta. The texture of the soup is thick enough to act as a sauce and you can enjoy the wonderful flavor twice.

3 pounds tomatoes, halved

5 garlic cloves, smashed

2 celery stalks, cut into 1-inch pieces

1 sweet onion, quartered

2 tablespoons extra-virgin olive oil

2 tablespoons apple cider vinegar

¼ teaspoon sea salt

3 cups chicken broth

½ cup heavy (whipping) cream

2 tablespoons chopped fresh basil

2 teaspoons chopped fresh oregano

1. Preheat the oven to 350°F.

2. In a large roasting pan, place the tomatoes cut-side down. Scatter the garlic, celery, and onion over the tomatoes. Drizzle with the olive oil and cider vinegar. Sprinkle with the sea salt.

3. Roast for 35 to 40 minutes, or until the tomatoes are tender. Cool for 15 minutes.

4. In a food processor or blender, purée the vegetables in small batches, adding the chicken broth in portions, as needed, to thin the texture.

5. Transfer the soup to a large nonreactive saucepan. Place it over medium heat and bring to a simmer.

6. Whisk in the cream, basil, and oregano. Serve hot.

 TIP When processing hot ingredients in a food processor or blender, use small batches. Remove the plug in the lid, cover the lid with a doubled clean cloth, and hold the lid down. The lid opening will allow the steam to escape, so the mixture won't overflow.

PER SERVING CALORIES: 153; FAT: 9G; SATURATED FAT: 1G;
PROTEIN: 5G; CARBS: 18G; SODIUM: 480MG; FIBER: 5G; SUGAR: 10G

OKTOBERFEST STEW

GLUTEN FREE

SERVES 4 • PREP TIME: 20 MINUTES • COOK TIME: 1 HOUR

This chunky, smoky stew is not for those who are counting calories. Caraway seeds—technically fruits of a parsley-like plant—are a common spice in German cuisine, where Oktoberfest originated. You might recognize their taste from some rye bread variations. If you do not have this spice in your pantry, substitute anise seeds with very little change in the character of the stew.

1 tablespoon extra-virgin olive oil	¼ teaspoon ground caraway seeds
1 sweet onion, chopped	1 cup dark beer
1 teaspoon minced garlic	2 cups chicken broth
1 (10-ounce) smoked sausage, cut into ¼-inch slices	2 Russet potatoes, peeled and cut into ½-inch cubes
2 cups shredded green cabbage	2 tablespoons apple cider vinegar
½ teaspoon freshly ground black pepper	2 tablespoons chopped fresh parsley

1. Place a large nonreactive saucepan over medium-high heat. Add the olive oil.

2. Add the onion and garlic. Sauté for about 3 minutes, or until translucent.

3. Add the sausage. Sauté for about 4 minutes, or until lightly browned.

4. Stir in the cabbage, pepper, and caraway. Sauté for 4 minutes to soften the cabbage.

5. Add the beer. Simmer the liquid for about 5 minutes, or until it is reduced by half.

6. Stir in the chicken broth and potatoes. Return the liquid to a simmer. Reduce the heat to low. Simmer for about 40 minutes, or until the potatoes are tender and the liquid is reduced by just over half. Stir in the cider vinegar.

7. Top with parsley and serve hot.

 TIP Beer is a common ingredient in stews and soups because it adds richness to the flavor and many important nutrients. Dark beer is an excellent source of health-boosting flavonoids. And studies, such as one conducted by the University of Wisconsin, have found that drinking dark beer in moderation can reduce the risk of heart disease.

PER SERVING CALORIES: 398; FAT: 24G; SATURATED FAT: 7G; PROTEIN: 17G; CARBS: 24G; SODIUM: 891MG; FIBER: 4G; SUGAR: 4G

MUSTARD CHICKEN SALAD

GLUTEN FREE **PALEO FRIENDLY** QUICK & EASY

SERVES 4 • PREP TIME: 20 MINUTES

Chicken, celery, and apple combine in a light mustard-citrus sauce for a dish that might remind you of the popular Waldorf salad. Dijon mustard, originally came only from an area in France near Burgundy; now any brand that follows the basic recipe for this condiment uses that designation. Traditional authentic Dijon mustard uses the sour juice of unripe grapes, verjuice, *rather than vinegar to produce the pleasing taste.*

For the dressing

2 tablespoons orange juice

2 tablespoons apple cider vinegar

2 tablespoons extra-virgin olive oil

1 tablespoon honey

1 teaspoon Dijon mustard

Juice of 1 lime

For the salad

2 (6-ounce) boneless skinless chicken breasts, cooked and shredded

2 celery stalks, chopped

1 apple, cored and chopped

1 small red bell pepper, seeded and cut into thin strips

1 scallion, white and green parts, sliced thin

¼ cup slivered almonds

2 tablespoons chopped fresh parsley

Freshly ground black pepper

2 cups shredded lettuce

To make the dressing

In a small nonreactive bowl, whisk together the orange juice, cider vinegar, olive oil, honey, Dijon mustard, and lime juice. Set aside.

To make the salad

1. In a large nonreactive bowl, toss together the chicken, celery, apple, bell pepper, scallion, almonds, and parsley until well mixed.

2. Add the dressing, and toss to coat.

3. Season with pepper.

4. Arrange the lettuce on 4 plates. Top each with one-fourth of the chicken salad.

PER SERVING CALORIES: 314; FAT: 17G; SATURATED FAT: 2G; PROTEIN: 27G; CARBS: 15G; SODIUM: 99MG; FIBER: 3G; SUGAR: 11G

SPICED CARROT SALAD

GLUTEN FREE **PALEO FRIENDLY** **QUICK & EASY** **VEGAN** **VEGETARIAN**

SERVES 4 • PREP TIME: 25 MINUTES • COOK TIME: 5 MINUTES

Carrots are in season in summer and early fall, so enjoy them in all your recipes while they are at their peak flavor. Carrots are known for their vision-protecting benefits, but this pretty root vegetable is also effective for helping prevent cardiovascular disease. The type of antioxidants in carrots, especially beta-carotene, is easily digested by the body and does not deteriorate—even after your carrots spend a week in the refrigerator.

---

8 carrots, cut into ½-inch chunks

½ cup golden raisins

¼ cup sliced almonds

2 tablespoons apple cider vinegar

1 tablespoon honey

1 tablespoon chopped fresh cilantro

1 tablespoon chopped fresh parsley

2 teaspoons extra-virgin olive oil

1 teaspoon minced garlic

½ teaspoon ground cumin

½ teaspoon ground coriander

Sea salt

Freshly ground black pepper

1. Fill a medium saucepan halfway with water. Place it over high heat. Bring to a boil.

2. Add the carrots. Blanch for about 4 minutes, or until crisp-tender. Drain and transfer to a large nonreactive bowl.

3. Add the raisins and almonds to the bowl. Toss to mix.

4. In a small nonreactive bowl, whisk together the cider vinegar, honey, cilantro, parsley, olive oil, garlic, cumin, and coriander.

5. Pour the dressing over the carrot mixture and toss to coat.

6. Season with sea salt and pepper.

7. Chill before serving.

 If you want to create a spectacular summer salad, get heirloom carrots in an assortment of colors. Carrots come in purple, yellow, red, and green hues and can sometimes be purchased in bags containing all shades for a reasonable cost. Blanch purple carrots only briefly, because the color can leach out.

PER SERVING CALORIES: 179; FAT: 6G; SATURATED FAT: 1G;
PROTEIN: 3G; CARBS: 32G; SODIUM: 88MG; FIBER: 5G; SUGAR: 21G

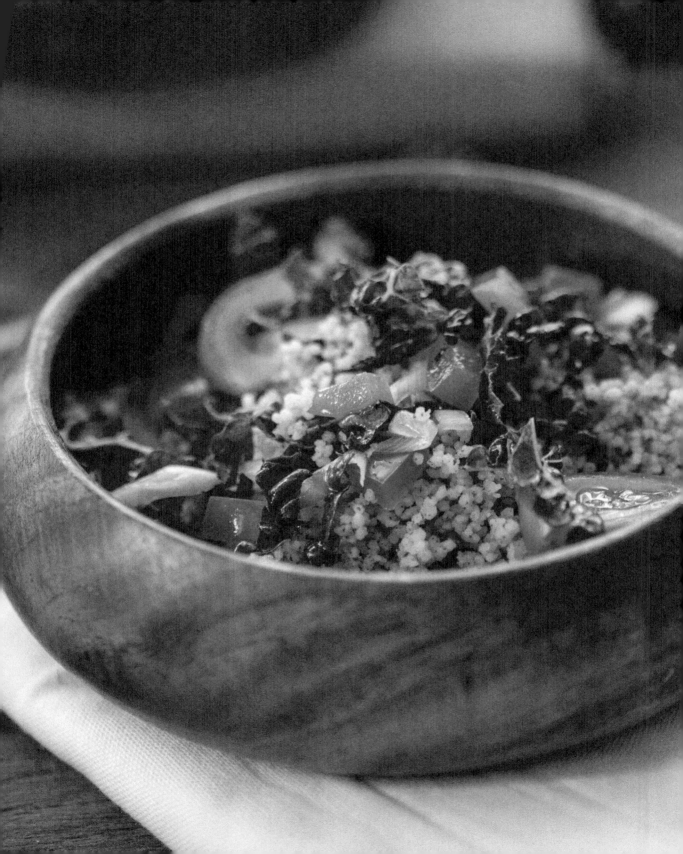

GREEK COUSCOUS SALAD

QUICK & EASY VEGETARIAN

SERVES 4 • PREP TIME: 20 MINUTES

Greek food seems somewhat unfinished without the addition of salty, firm, feta cheese—which is no surprise considering it represents about 70 percent of the cheese consumed in Greece. In this recipe, the cheese is optional, but it certainly adds a lovely flavor and appearance to the dish. Traditional feta consists of a combination of goat's milk and sheep's milk from animals raised in certain areas of the country. The animal breed, grazing conditions, region, and type of brine used all combine to create cheeses that range from mild and creamy to robust and firm.

For the dressing
¼ cup apple cider vinegar
2 tablespoons chopped fresh basil
1 teaspoon chopped fresh oregano
Pinch sea salt
Pinch freshly ground black pepper
½ cup extra-virgin olive oil

For the salad
3 cups cooked couscous
1 small red onion, chopped
1 red bell pepper, seeded and diced
2 cups halved cherry tomatoes
1 cup shredded kale
1 scallion, white and green parts, chopped
½ cup crumbled feta cheese (optional)

To make the dressing

1. In a small nonreactive bowl, whisk together the cider vinegar, basil, oregano, sea salt, and pepper until combined.

2. Slowly whisk in the olive oil until the dressing is emulsified. Set aside.

To make the salad

1. In a large nonreactive bowl, stir together the couscous, onion, bell pepper, tomatoes, and kale until well mixed.

2. Pour the dressing over the salad, and toss to combine.

3. Top with the scallion and serve.

 TIP Couscous is one of the easiest pasta products to cook and can be made several days ahead for cold salads and sides. Couscous cooks in a 1:1 ratio with liquid. One cup of dried couscous produces about 4 cups cooked. For this recipe, use about ¾ cup dried couscous to get the right amount.

PER SERVING CALORIES: 403; FAT: 28G; SATURATED FAT: 6G;
PROTEIN: 7G; CARBS: 32G; SODIUM: 225MG; FIBER: 3G; SUGAR: 3G

GRILLED VEGETABLE PASTA SALAD

QUICK & EASY VEGETARIAN

SERVES 4 • PREP TIME: 20 MINUTES • COOK TIME: 10 MINUTES

This colorful, filling salad might become your "go to" dish on balmy summer days, either as an accompaniment to grilled meats or as a light meal by itself. Portobello mushrooms are frequently used as a meat substitute because their texture is dense and they taste fabulous with many other ingredients. If you don't like the dark color that portobellos add to a recipe, remove the black gills with a spoon before using. For grilling the vegetables, you'll want to use a grilling basket that will hold small pieces so they won't fall through the grill.

5 tablespoons extra-virgin olive oil, divided

½ small red onion, sliced

1 green zucchini, sliced lengthwise into ¼-inch strips

1 yellow zucchini, slice lengthwise into ¼-inch strips

1 red bell pepper, seeded and halved

3 large portobello mushrooms, stemmed and wiped cleaned

10 asparagus spears, woody ends trimmed

1 cup cherry tomatoes, halved

5 cups cooked farfalle pasta

Juice of 1 lemon

2 tablespoons apple cider vinegar

Freshly ground black pepper

½ cup crumbled soft goat cheese (chèvre)

2 tablespoons chopped fresh basil

1. Preheat the grill to medium heat.

2. In a large bowl, mix together 1 tablespoon of the olive oil, the red onion, green zucchini, yellow zucchini, bell pepper, mushrooms, and asparagus.

3. Put the vegetables in a grilling basket and put on the grill. Cook for about 10 minutes, or until tender and slightly charred. Cool the vegetables slightly and chop them coarsely.

4. In a large nonreactive bowl, combine the cherry tomatoes, cooked pasta, and chopped vegetables.

5. In a small nonreactive bowl, whisk together the remaining 4 tablespoons olive oil, the lemon juice, and the cider vinegar.

6. Pour the dressing over the salad and toss to coat. Season the salad with pepper.

7. Top the salad with the crumbled goat cheese and chopped basil, and serve.

PER SERVING CALORIES: 373; FAT: 24G; SATURATED FAT: 5G;
PROTEIN: 14G; CARBS: 30G; SODIUM: 68MG; FIBER: 5G; SUGAR: 6G

POTATO SALAD WITH HOT BACON DRESSING

GLUTEN FREE

SERVES 4 • PREP TIME: 20 MINUTES • COOK TIME: 25 MINUTES

Most picnickers associate potato salad with a cold mayonnaise-drenched dish enhanced with chopped hard-boiled eggs and a sprinkle of paprika. Potato salad can also be warm, vinegary, and studded with crisp bacon bits and pungent scallions. Hot potato salad originated before the cold version hundreds of years before refrigeration was common. This salad is particularly delicious when served alongside barbecued ribs or chicken.

2 pounds red fingerling potatoes, scrubbed

½ teaspoon sea salt

2 scallions, green and white parts, chopped

10 bacon slices, diced

2 teaspoons minced garlic

⅓ cup apple cider vinegar

3 tablespoons sugar

1 tablespoon Dijon mustard

Sea salt

Freshly ground black pepper

3 tablespoons chopped fresh parsley

1. Place the potatoes in a large pot. Fill the pot with enough cold water to cover the potatoes by 3 inches. Add the sea salt.

2. Place the pot over high heat and bring to a boil. Reduce the heat to low. Simmer the potatoes for about 15 minutes, or until just fork-tender.

3. Drain the potatoes. Set aside for about 15 minutes, or until cool enough to handle. Over a large nonreactive bowl, cut the potatoes into ½-inch chunks. Add the scallions and set aside.

4. Place a medium nonreactive saucepan over medium heat. Add the bacon. Cook for about 6 minutes, stirring occasionally, until crispy. With a slotted spoon, transfer the bacon to the bowl with the potatoes.

5. Return the saucepan with the bacon fat to the stove, still over medium heat. Whisk in the garlic, cider vinegar, sugar, and Dijon mustard. Bring to a simmer. Cook for 2 minutes.

6. Pour the dressing over the potatoes and gently toss to combine.

7. Season with sea salt and pepper. Top with the parsley and serve warm.

PER SERVING CALORIES: 267; FAT: 2G; SATURATED FAT: 1G;
PROTEIN: 10G; CARBS: 50G; SODIUM: 830MG; FIBER: 4G; SUGAR: 11G

FENNEL-JICAMA SALAD

GLUTEN FREE **PALEO FRIENDLY QUICK & EASY VEGAN** VEGETARIAN

SERVES 4 • PREP TIME: 30 MINUTES

Jicama looks like a large oval potato, but it has a thick, tough, inedible skin that needs to be removed. Inside is snowy, crisp flesh that tastes like a cross between a pear and turnip. Jicama is low in calories and the body does not metabolize its fiber. Jicama is an excellent source of vitamin C, potassium, and magnesium.

For the dressing

¼ cup extra-virgin olive oil

3 tablespoons apple cider vinegar

1 tablespoon chopped fresh basil

1 teaspoon honey

For the salad

1 fennel bulb, well washed and shredded

1 jicama, peeled and shredded

1 McIntosh apple, cored and diced

3 large radishes, sliced thin

2 cups julienned arugula

½ cup dried cranberries

1 tablespoon freshly squeezed lemon juice

Sea salt

Freshly ground black pepper

1 scallion, green and white parts, chopped

To make the dressing

In a small nonreactive bowl, whisk together the olive oil, cider vinegar, basil, and honey. Set aside.

To make the salad

1. In a large nonreactive bowl, toss together the fennel, jicama, apple, radishes, arugula, cranberries, and lemon juice until mixed.

2. Add the dressing to the salad and toss to combine.

3. Season with sea salt and pepper. Top with the scallion and serve.

PER SERVING CALORIES: 232; FAT: 13G; SATURATED FAT: 2G; PROTEIN: 2G; CARBS: 29G; SODIUM: 44MG; FIBER: 12G; SUGAR: 10G

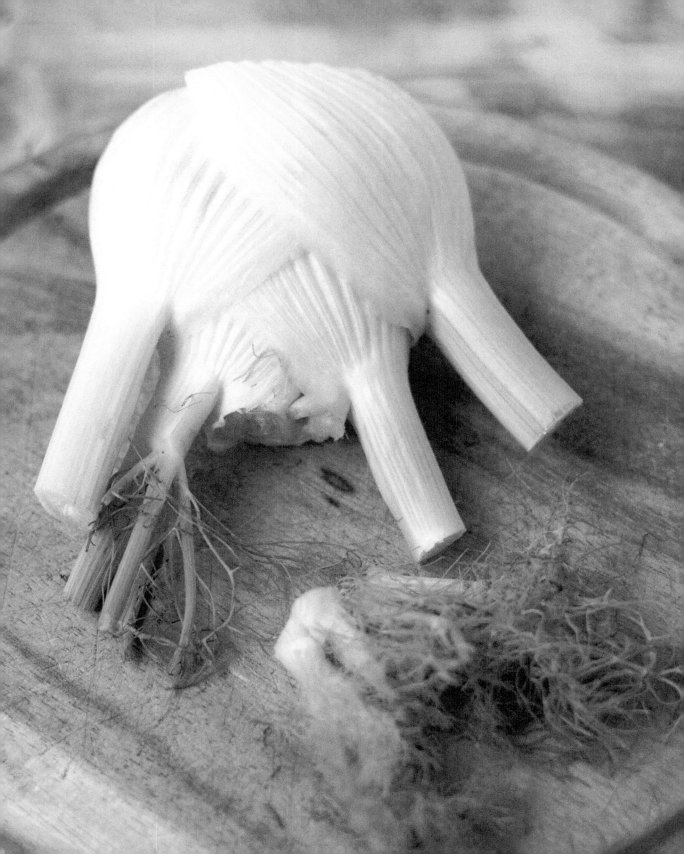

ASIAN ASPARAGUS SALAD

GLUTEN FREE **QUICK & EASY** **VEGAN** VEGETARIAN

SERVES 4 • PREP TIME: 30 MINUTES

Peeling asparagus into ribbons reveals a lighter interior color surrounded by the outside's deep green—transforming the simple spear into an elegant ingredient. Pick spears that are about ½ inch in diameter. Larger ones tend to be bitter, and thinner, tender spears will break when you peel them.

For the dressing

2 tablespoons sesame oil

2 tablespoons apple cider vinegar

1 tablespoon honey

1 tablespoon chopped fresh cilantro

1 teaspoon grated peeled fresh ginger

1 teaspoon chili paste

½ teaspoon minced garlic

Zest of 1 lime

Juice of 1 lime

For the salad

20 asparagus spears, woody ends trimmed, peeled into long, thin ribbons with a vegetable peeler

1 cup shredded stemmed kale, thoroughly washed

2 scallions, sliced very thin

½ cup chopped cashews

To make the dressing

In a small nonreactive bowl, whisk together the sesame oil, cider vinegar, honey, cilantro, ginger, chili paste, garlic, lime zest, and lime juice until well blended. Set aside.

To make the salad

1. In a large nonreactive bowl, combine the asparagus ribbons, kale, and scallions.

2. Pour the dressing over the vegetables and toss to coat.

3. Top with the cashews and serve.

PER SERVING CALORIES: 217; FAT: 15G; SATURATED FAT: 3G; PROTEIN: 6G; CARBS: 18G; SODIUM: 30G; FIBER: 4G; SUGAR: 8G

WATERMELON-TOMATO SALAD

GLUTEN FREE **QUICK & EASY** VEGETARIAN

SERVES 4 • PREP TIME: 30 MINUTES, PLUS 3 HOURS CHILLING TIME

Fresh herbs enhance foods' flavors and can also add visual impact to a dish. The mint and cilantro in this recipe do both. Mint has one of the most popular flavor profiles in the world and can be found in beverages, candy, desserts, main courses, and salads across many cultures. Mint has one of the highest antioxidant contents of any food and can help relieve allergies, fight the common cold, and calm indigestion.

For the dressing

3 tablespoons apple cider vinegar

2 tablespoons extra-virgin olive oil

Pinch of freshly ground black pepper

For the salad

4 cups diced seedless watermelon

2 cups halved cherry tomatoes

1 scallion, green and white parts, chopped

½ English cucumber, diced

½ cup crumbled feta cheese

¼ cup chopped fresh mint

1 tablespoon chopped fresh cilantro

To make the dressing

In a small nonreactive bowl, whisk together the cider vinegar, olive oil, and pepper. Set aside.

To make the salad

1. In a large nonreactive bowl, toss together the watermelon, tomatoes, scallion, cucumber, feta cheese, mint, and cilantro.

2. Add the dressing to the salad and toss to mix well.

3. Chill completely, for about 3 hours, and serve.

 Most of watermelon's nutritional benefits are found in the pale green layer between the rind and juicy red flesh. With a vegetable peeler, peel the rind off the melon but leave most of the pale green middle layer intact. When you cut it into chunks for the salad, the color variation will make a beautiful presentation and you will keep all the health benefits of the watermelon.

PER SERVING CALORIES: 167; FAT: 11G; SATURATED FAT: 4G; PROTEIN: 4G; CARBS: 14G; SODIUM: 215MG; FIBER: 1G; SUGAR: 11G

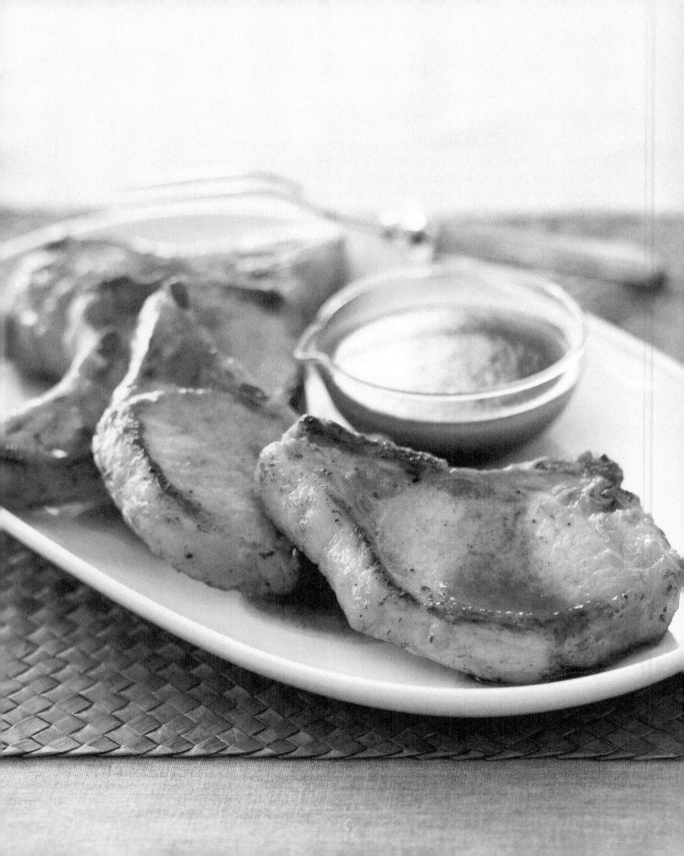

Chapter Ten

ENTRÉES

158   Tahini Curry Noodle Bowl

160   Wild Rice Bowl

161   Wheat Berry–Stuffed Tomatoes

162   Scallops with Bacon Cream Sauce

163   Herb-Marinated Halibut

165   Chicken Pot Pie

167   Maple Salmon Packets with Asian Vegetables

168   Honey Tomato Chicken Drumsticks

169   Chinese Chicken Lettuce Wraps

170   Linguine Carbonara

172   Chili Dry Rub Pork Ribs

174   Maple Cider Pork Chops

175   Spicy Sloppy Joes

176   Flank Steak with Citrus Marinade

177   Traditional Sauerbraten

TAHINI CURRY NOODLE BOWL

GLUTEN FREE **QUICK & EASY VEGAN** VEGETARIAN

SERVES 4 • PREP TIME: 15 MINUTES • COOK TIME: 10 MINUTES

Coconut milk is made by grating fresh coconut, combining it with water, and squeezing the mixture through cheesecloth. Coconut milk is thick or thin depending on the product and whether it is boxed or canned. This recipe uses the thick, canned coconut milk rather than the variety in a carton found at your local grocery store. In cans, the coconut milk tends to separate, so be sure to stir the can contents before measuring it out.

For the sauce

¼ cup tahini

¼ cup canned coconut milk

2 tablespoons apple cider vinegar

1 tablespoon extra-virgin olive oil

2 teaspoons curry powder

1½ teaspoons ground cumin

1 teaspoon ground coriander

1 teaspoon grated peeled fresh ginger

½ teaspoon ground turmeric

½ teaspoon freshly ground black pepper

For the noodle bowl

1 (8-ounce / 225-gram) package rice noodles

2 carrots, shredded

1 red bell pepper, seeded and diced

1 cup fresh snow peas, stems and strings removed, julienned

1 cup stemmed shredded kale, thoroughly washed

3 tablespoons chopped fresh cilantro

To make the sauce

1. In a blender, combine the tahini, coconut milk, cider vinegar, olive oil, curry powder, cumin, coriander, ginger, turmeric, and black pepper.

2. Pulse until smooth and well mixed. Set aside.

To make the noodle bowl

1. Place the rice noodles in a large nonreactive bowl.

2. Bring a large pot of water to a boil over high heat. Pour the boiling water over the rice noodles to cover completely. Let sit for about 10 minutes, stirring 3 to 4 times, until tender and cooked. Drain the noodles and return them to the bowl.

3. Add the carrots, bell pepper, snow peas, kale, and cilantro. Toss to combine.

4. Add the dressing. Toss to coat.

5. Serve immediately or refrigerate in a sealed container for up to 2 days.

 The best type of tahini to purchase is labeled unhulled because it is made from whole, intact sesame seeds, which preserves all the nutritional benefits. This fragrant paste is high in vitamin E and most of the B vitamins, as well as potassium and iron. Tahini is also a fabulous source of protein and healthy unsaturated fat.

PER SERVING CALORIES: 419; FAT: 16G; SATURATED FAT: 5G; PROTEIN: 7G; CARBS: 62G; SODIUM: 157MG; FIBER: 6G; SUGAR: 5G

WILD RICE BOWL

GLUTEN FREE **VEGAN** VEGETARIAN

SERVES 4 • PREP TIME: 25 MINUTES • COOK TIME: 50 MINUTES

Cranberries add an appealing tartness to this wild rice mixture, along with the apple cider vinegar. Cranberries—an excellent source of protein, fiber, and vitamins A, C, E, and K can also boost the immune system, which is why they make such an effective treatment for urinary tract infections.

For the sauce

¼ cup apple cider vinegar

Juice of 1 lime

2 tablespoons honey

1 tablespoon extra-virgin olive oil

3 tablespoons chopped fresh cilantro

1 teaspoon grated peeled fresh ginger

¼ teaspoon garlic powder

For the rice bowl

1½ cups wild rice

2 cups shredded napa cabbage

1 carrot, shredded

1 red bell pepper, seeded and chopped

1 jicama, peeled and shredded

1 cup dried cranberries

½ cup chopped pistachios

2 scallions, white and green parts, sliced thin on a diagonal

To make the sauce

In a blender, combine the cider vinegar, lime juice, honey, olive oil, cilantro, ginger, and garlic powder. Blend until smooth. Set aside.

To make the rice bowl

1. In a medium saucepan, combine the wild rice with enough cold water to cover by about 3 inches. Place the pan over medium-high heat and bring to a boil. Reduce the heat to low. Cover and simmer the rice for about 50 minutes, or until tender.

2. Drain the rice and transfer it to a large nonreactive bowl. Add the cabbage, carrot, bell pepper, jicama, cranberries, and pistachios. Toss to combine.

3. Pour the dressing over the rice and vegetables. Stir to coat.

4. Top with the scallions and serve.

 TIP Wild rice actually is a type of grass. It is easy to digest and is often tolerated by people who are gluten intolerant.

PER SERVING CALORIES: 468; FAT: 12G; SATURATED FAT: 2G; PROTEIN: 14G; CARBS: 80G; SODIUM: 47MG; FIBER: 16G; SUGAR: 18G

WHEAT BERRY–STUFFED TOMATOES

GLUTEN FREE **VEGETARIAN**

SERVES 4 • PREP TIME: 15 MINUTES, PLUS 30 MINUTES DRAINING TIME • COOK TIME: 50 MINUTES

Vegetables make naturally beautiful containers for an assortment of fillings. The tomatoes could be replaced with bell peppers, squash, or zucchini. You can prepare this dish completely and refrigerate it until you're ready to bake it.

Butter, for the baking dish

4 large firm tomatoes

Sea salt

1 teaspoon extra-virgin olive oil

1 yellow bell pepper, seeded and chopped

½ sweet onion, chopped

1 teaspoon minced garlic

2 tablespoons apple cider vinegar

1½ cups cooked wheat berries

2 tablespoons chopped fresh basil

2 tablespoons chopped fresh parsley

Freshly ground black pepper

¼ cup crumbled chèvre goat cheese

1. Preheat the oven to 350°F. Lightly butter an 8-by-8-inch baking dish.

2. Slice the tops off the tomatoes and scoop out the pulp, leaving the outside shell intact. Chop the pulp coarsely and transfer it to a bowl. Set aside.

3. Sprinkle the inside of the tomatoes with ½ teaspoon of the sea salt. Place them upside down on paper towels to drain for 30 minutes.

4. Add the olive oil to a medium nonreactive skillet set over medium heat. Add the bell pepper, onion, and garlic. Sauté for about 4 minutes, or until softened.

5. Stir in the reserved tomato pulp and cider vinegar. Bring to a boil. Reduce the heat to low and simmer for 10 minutes, stirring occasionally.

6. Add the wheat berries, basil, and parsley to the skillet. Cook for 5 minutes, or until all ingredients are heated through. Remove the filling from the heat and season with sea salt and pepper.

7. Place the drained tomato shells in the prepared baking dish. Spoon one-fourth of the filling into each.

8. Bake for about 25 minutes, or until the filling is hot and the tomatoes are softened and lightly browned.

9. Top each tomato with about 1 tablespoon of the chèvre and bake for 5 more minutes. Serve warm.

PER SERVING CALORIES: 173; FAT: 5G; SATURATED FAT: 2G; PROTEIN: 7G; CARBS: 28G; SODIUM: 277MG; FIBER: 4G; SUGAR: 7G

SCALLOPS WITH BACON CREAM SAUCE

GLUTEN FREE **QUICK & EASY**

SERVES 4 • PREP TIME: 10 MINUTES • COOK TIME: 20 MINUTES

Scallops need to be examined closely before using, to ensure a superior result. Run each scallop under cold water while touching the entire surface to rub away any grit or sand. Carefully feel the sides of the scallop for the remaining side muscle and remove it. These sections are tougher and the fibers run opposite to the grain.

12 jumbo sea scallops, washed, trimmed and patted dry

Sea salt

Freshly ground black pepper

4 bacon slices, chopped

5 ounces oyster mushrooms

½ teaspoon minced garlic

½ cup heavy (whipping) cream

2 tablespoons apple cider vinegar

1 tablespoon honey

2 teaspoons chopped fresh thyme

1 tablespoon butter

1. Lightly season the scallops on both sides with sea salt and pepper. Set aside.

2. Place a large nonreactive skillet over medium-high heat. Add the bacon. Sauté for about 5 minutes, or until crispy. With a slotted spoon, transfer the bacon to a small bowl.

3. In the bacon fat remaining in the skillet, sauté the mushrooms and garlic for about 4 minutes, or until the mushrooms are golden brown.

4. Stir in the reserved bacon, heavy cream, cider vinegar, honey, and thyme. Cook for about 2 minutes, or until the sauce is thick. Remove from the heat and set aside.

5. Place another large skillet over medium-high heat and melt the butter.

6. When placing the scallops in the skillet, the first one should sizzle when it touches the hot butter. If not, wait until the butter is hot. Place the scallops in a single layer without crowding the pan. Cook for 2 minutes and then turn them over. Cook for 3 minutes more on the second side, or until both sides are seared and the scallops are opaque.

7. Evenly divide the sauce among 4 plates and top each with 3 scallops.

8. Serve immediately.

PER SERVING CALORIES: 270; FAT: 14G; SATURATED FAT: 8G; PROTEIN: 23G; CARBS: 12G; SODIUM: 522MG; FIBER: 1G; SUGAR: 6G

HERB-MARINATED HALIBUT

GLUTEN FREE **PALEO FRIENDLY**

SERVES 4 • PREP TIME: 10 MINUTES, PLUS 1 HOUR MARINATING TIME • COOK TIME: 20 MINUTES

If you don't cook fish often, you likely choose frozen when you do. But fresh products can be simple to pick and have a superior texture. Advances in refrigeration have increased the availability of fresh fish, and farmed fish has dropped the price of many species, making fish a viable choice even for families on modest budgets. This recipe can be made with either fresh or frozen fish.

½ cup extra-virgin olive oil

¼ cup apple cider vinegar

¼ cup freshly squeezed lemon juice

1 tablespoon chopped fresh basil

1 tablespoon chopped fresh oregano

1 teaspoon chopped fresh thyme

1 teaspoon minced garlic

¼ teaspoon freshly ground black pepper

4 (6-ounce) halibut fillets

Lime wedges, for garnish

1. In a medium nonreactive bowl, whisk together the olive oil, cider vinegar, lemon juice, basil, oregano, thyme, garlic, and black pepper until well blended.

2. Add the fish fillets, and turn to coat. Cover the bowl with plastic wrap, and marinate the fish in the refrigerator for 1 hour.

3. Preheat the oven to 350°F. Line a baking sheet with aluminum foil.

4. Transfer the fish to the prepared baking sheet. Bake for 18 to 20 minutes, or until the fish flakes easily when pressed lightly.

5. Garnish with lime wedges and serve.

PER SERVING CALORIES: 364; FAT: 26G; SATURATED FAT: 4G;
PROTEIN: 30G; CARBS: 2G; SODIUM: 87MG; FIBER: 1G; SUGAR: 0G

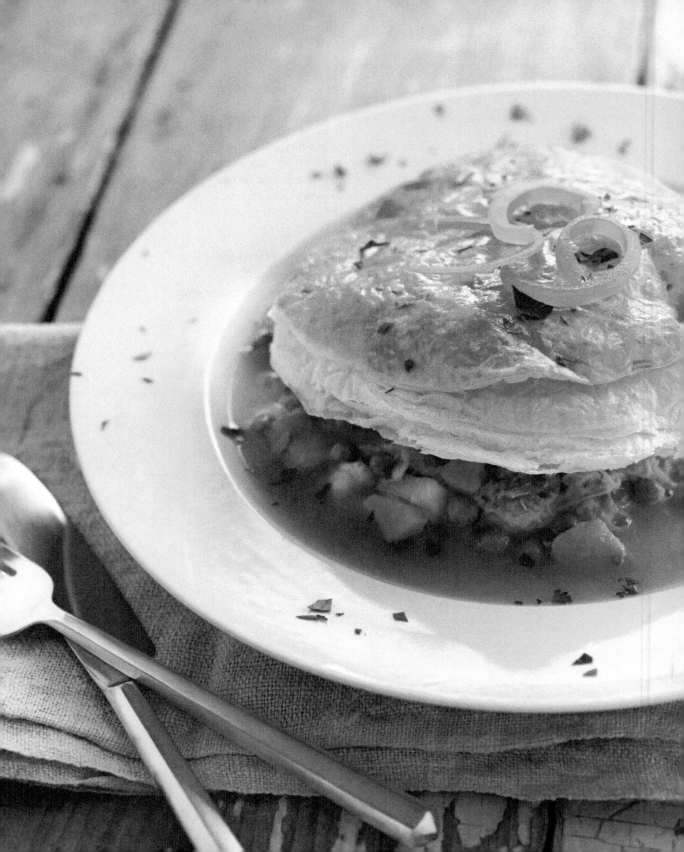

CHICKEN POT PIE

SERVES 8 • PREP TIME: 30 MINUTES • COOK TIME: 40 MINUTES

Chicken pot pie is often made in a baked pie crust, but this version is topped with a puff pastry baked to a beautiful golden brown. The filling will be bubbly hot when you spoon it on the plate and it will soak into the bottom of each crispy topping.

For the filling

2 potatoes, peeled and diced

1 large carrot, diced

3 tablespoons butter

1 sweet onion, chopped

2 teaspoons minced garlic

3 tablespoons all-purpose flour

2 cups chicken broth

2 tablespoons apple cider vinegar

1 teaspoon chopped fresh thyme

1 teaspoon chopped fresh tarragon

Sea salt

Freshly ground black pepper

3 cups diced cooked chicken

1 cup frozen peas

For the topping

1 (17-ounce) package puff pastry, thawed

Flour for dusting

To make the filling

1. Fill a medium saucepan three-fourths full of water. Place it over high heat and bring to a boil. Add the potatoes and carrot. Blanch for about 6 minutes, or until just tender. Drain the vegetables and set aside.

2. In a large saucepan set over medium-high heat, melt the butter. Add the onion and garlic. Sauté for about 3 minutes, or until translucent.

3. Whisk in the flour to form a paste. Cook for about 4 minutes, whisking constantly, until the flour browns.

4. Pour in the chicken broth and apple cider vinegar, whisking constantly. Cook for about 3 minutes, whisking constantly, until the sauce thickens.

5. Remove the saucepan from the heat and stir in the thyme and tarragon. Season with sea salt and pepper. Stir in the potatoes, carrot, chicken, and peas.

6. Keep the chicken mixture in the saucepan on low heat to keep it warm while baking the topping.

continued

To make the topping

1. Preheat the oven to 400°F.

2. Lightly flour your work surface and unfold your thawed puff pastry sheet.

3. Roll the puff pastry out on the floured surface until it is about ½ inch thick.

4. Use a round cutter or a 4-inch water glass to cut out 8 rounds in the pasty dough.

5. Transfer the rounds to a baking sheet.

6. Bake the puff pastry until it is golden brown and puffed, about 15 minutes.

7. Spoon the chicken mixture into a bowl and top each portion with a baked puff pastry round. Serve hot.

PER SERVING CALORIES: 433; FAT: 22G; SATURATED FAT: 7G;
PROTEIN: 22G; CARBS: 35G; SODIUM: 384MG; FIBER: 4G; SUGAR: 3G

MAPLE SALMON PACKETS WITH ASIAN VEGETABLES

GLUTEN FREE **PALEO FRIENDLY** QUICK & EASY

SERVES 4 • PREP TIME: 20 MINUTES • COOK TIME: 15 MINUTES

Salmon is the fish most commonly prepared at home. Salmon flesh can vary extensively in color depending on whether it is farmed or wild. Farmed salmon has a pale pink hue, unless deliberately dyed, and wild salmon is a gorgeous rich, deep red. Choose your salmon depending on what your budget allows.

---

8 small bok choy, sliced

1 cup bean sprouts

1 cup baby corn, cut into 1-inch pieces

1 carrot, peeled and sliced

2 scallions, green and white parts, chopped

4 (6-ounce) boneless skinless salmon fillets

¼ cup maple syrup

2 tablespoons low-sodium tamari sauce

2 tablespoons apple cider vinegar

1 teaspoon grated peeled fresh ginger

Pinch red pepper flakes

1. Preheat the oven to 400°F.

2. Place 4 (12-by-12-inch) aluminum foil squares on a work surface.

3. In the center of each square, place one-fourth of the bok choy, ¼ cup bean sprouts, ¼ cup baby corn, one-fourth of the carrot, and one-fourth of the scallions. Top each with 1 salmon fillet.

4. In a small nonreactive bowl, stir together the maple syrup, tamari sauce, cider vinegar, ginger, and red pepper flakes. Drizzle evenly over the fish. Fold the foil up around the fish to form loosely sealed packets.

5. Transfer the salmon packets to a baking sheet. Bake for about 15 minutes, or until the fish is just cooked through.

6. Open the packets carefully to avoid the escaping steam and serve.

PER SERVING CALORIES: 363; FAT: 11G; SATURATED FAT: 2G;
PROTEIN: 39G; CARBS: 30G; SODIUM: 532MG; FIBER: 4G; SUGAR: 14G

HONEY TOMATO CHICKEN DRUMSTICKS

GLUTEN FREE (SEE TIP) **PALEO FRIENDLY**

SERVES 4 • PREP TIME: 10 MINUTES, PLUS 6 HOURS MARINATING TIME • COOK TIME: 15 MINUTES

Garlic plays an important role in the complex, almost luxurious, flavor of this sauce. This popular allium vegetable has more than 70 phytochemicals, which can help fight the common cold, prevent many cancers, and lower blood pressure. Garlic is high in manganese, calcium, selenium, and fiber, as well as vitamins B_1, B_6, and C.

1 (6-ounce) can tomato paste	1 teaspoon minced garlic
2 tablespoons honey	1 teaspoon Worcestershire sauce (see Tip)
2 tablespoons apple cider vinegar	8 (4-ounce) chicken drumsticks
2 teaspoons Dijon mustard	Sea salt
2 teaspoons extra-virgin olive oil	Freshly ground black pepper

1. In a large nonreactive bowl, stir together the tomato paste, honey, cider vinegar, Dijon mustard, olive oil, garlic, and Worcestershire sauce.

2. With a sharp knife, make 3 slashes in each drumstick. Season them with sea salt and pepper.

3. Add the drumsticks to the marinade and turn to coat. Cover with plastic wrap. Refrigerate for 6 hours to marinate.

4. Preheat the grill to medium-high.

5. Remove the drumsticks from the marinade and shake off the excess.

6. Grill the chicken for about 15 minutes, turning once halfway through, until it is cooked through.

 TIP This recipe is only considered gluten free if the Worcestershire sauce you use is gluten free. Check the label for rye, barley, malt vinegar, soy sauce, or "natural flavorings." These ingredients are not acceptable on a gluten-free diet.

PER SERVING CALORIES: 303; FAT: 8G; SATURATED FAT: 2G; PROTEIN: 28G; CARBS: 30G; SODIUM: 177MG; FIBER: 6G; SUGAR: 21G

CHINESE CHICKEN LETTUCE WRAPS

GLUTEN FREE **PALEO FRIENDLY**

SERVES 4 • PREP TIME: 20 MINUTES • COOK TIME: 15 MINUTES

Save some time when creating healthy meals by poaching or roasting a batch of chicken breasts at the beginning of the week. You can use them in soups, main courses, and dishes such as these spicy wraps. Refrigerate the cooked chicken breasts in resealable plastic bags. They will keep in the refrigerator up to 5 days.

For the sauce

3 tablespoons apple cider vinegar

1 tablespoon water

2 teaspoons sugar

2 teaspoons cornstarch

1 teaspoon grated peeled fresh ginger

1 teaspoon hoisin sauce

1 teaspoon soy sauce

½ teaspoon minced garlic

For the chicken

1 teaspoon extra-virgin olive oil

8 ounces cooked chicken breast, cut into thin strips

1 large carrot, julienned

1 red bell pepper, julienned

½ cup bean sprouts

½ cup snow peas, stems and strings removed, julienned

2 scallions, green and white parts, sliced

8 to 12 large Boston lettuce leaves

To make the sauce

In a small nonreactive bowl, whisk together the cider vinegar, water, sugar, cornstarch, ginger, hoisin sauce, soy sauce, and garlic. Set aside.

To make the chicken

1. Place a large nonreactive skillet over medium-high heat. Add the olive oil.

2. Add the chicken, carrot, bell pepper, bean sprouts, snow peas, and scallions to the skillet. Sauté for about 5 minutes, or until vegetables are crisp-tender.

3. Stir in the sauce. Cook for about 4 minutes, stirring constantly, until thickened.

4. Scoop the filling into a small serving bowl and place on a platter, surrounded by the lettuce leaves. Pass at the table, allowing each person to make their own wraps.

PER SERVING CALORIES: 158; FAT: 4G; SATURATED FAT: 0G; PROTEIN: 21G; CARBS: 11G; SODIUM: 180MG; FIBER: 2G; SUGAR: 6G

LINGUINE CARBONARA

QUICK & EASY

MAKES 4 SERVINGS • PREP TIME: 10 MINUTES • COOK TIME: 20 MINUTES

One of the more popular theories about carbonara sauce and its origins credits American soldiers after World War II. Away from home and seeking the comfort of familiar foods, and mistaking guanciale (cured pork jowl) for bacon, they requested it be added to this egg-sauced dish. Carbonara sauce can be made with Parma ham, prosciutto, or pancetta, if you want a sauce with even more flavor.

---

4 bacon slices, chopped

1 hot Italian sausage, cooked and cut into slices

1 tablespoon minced garlic

½ cup sliced mushrooms

½ cup dry white wine

1 (8-ounce) package linguine

4 eggs

½ cup heavy (whipping) cream

2 tablespoons apple cider vinegar

¼ cup fresh basil (optional)

¼ cup chopped fresh parsley (optional)

Pinch of red pepper flakes

½ cup spinach

½ cup grated Parmesan cheese

Sea salt

Freshly ground black pepper

1. In a large nonreactive skillet set over medium-high heat, cook the bacon for about 4 minutes, or until crispy.

2. Add the sausage, garlic, and mushrooms. Sauté for 4 minutes. Transfer the bacon, sausage, garlic, and mushrooms to a plate. Wipe the bacon fat from the skillet with a paper towel. Place the skillet back over medium-high heat.

3. Add the white wine, bacon, sausage, garlic, and mushrooms. Bring to a boil. Remove from the heat and set aside while you cook the linguine.

4. Cook the linguine according to package directions. Drain and set aside.

5. In a small nonreactive bowl, whisk together the eggs, heavy cream, cider vinegar, basil (optional), and parsley (optional).

6. Pour the egg mixture into the skillet with the bacon. Place the skillet over medium heat and whisk for about 5 minutes, or until the mixture thickens.

7. Whisk in the spinach and Parmesan cheese. Simmer for 1 minute. Season with sea salt and pepper.

8. Remove the sauce from the heat. Add the cooked linguine and toss to coat.

PER SERVING CALORIES: 448; FAT: 22G; SATURATED FAT: 10G; PROTEIN: 23G; CARBS: 35G; SODIUM: 506MG; FIBER: 0G; SUGAR: 1G

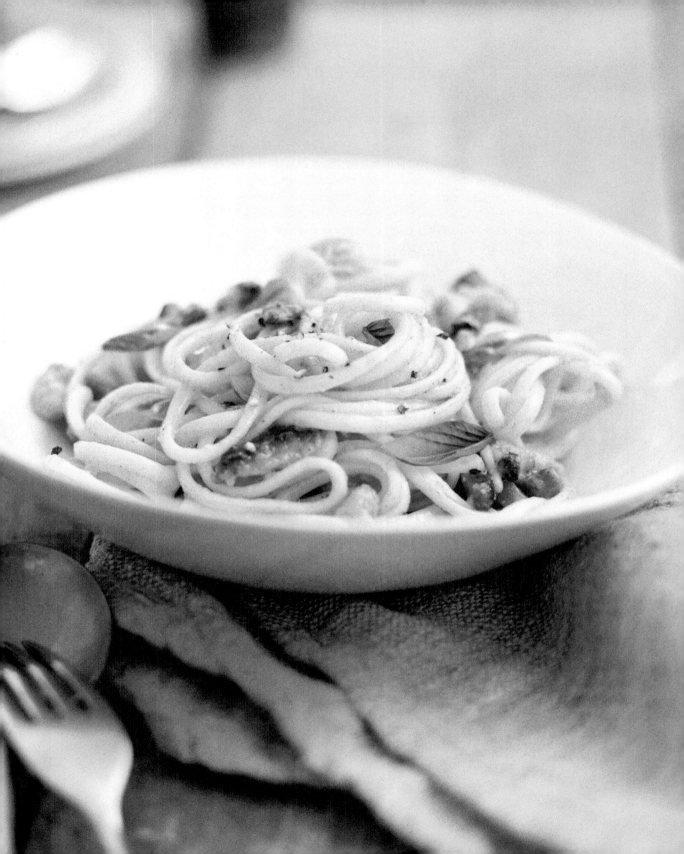

CHILI DRY RUB PORK RIBS

GLUTEN FREE **PALEO FRIENDLY**

SERVES 4 • PREP TIME: 25 MINUTES • COOK TIME: 3 HOURS

Great ribs are serious business for many chefs and amateur cooks. Rubs, sauces, mops, smoke, cooking methods, and the types of ribs used are all subject to intense debate. There are two cuts of pork ribs that could be used for this dish, depending on your preference: baby back ribs, which come from the area where the ribs meet the spine, or spare ribs. Baby back ribs, which are shorter than spare ribs, are very lean and tender, so they can be more expensive than the fattier spare ribs.

For the dry rub

½ cup chili powder

¼ cup ground cumin

2 tablespoons garlic powder

2 tablespoons onion powder

1 teaspoon sea salt

For the ribs

2 full racks pork baby back ribs

¼ cup prepared (yellow) mustard

For the mop sauce

½ cup apple cider vinegar

2 tablespoons water

2 tablespoons honey

2 tablespoons Dijon mustard

To make the dry rub

In a small bowl, stir together the chili powder, cumin, garlic powder, onion powder, and sea salt. Set aside.

To make the ribs

1. Preheat the oven to 350°F.
2. Brush the ribs with a thin layer of the prepared yellow mustard.
3. Liberally press the dry rub all over both sides of the ribs.
4. Wrap each rib rack in aluminum foil and place on a baking sheet.
5. Bake for 2 hours. Remove from the oven and cool.
6. Refrigerate the ribs, wrapped, until you want to finish them on the grill.

To make the mop sauce

In a small nonreactive bowl, stir together the cider vinegar, water, honey, and Dijon mustard.

To finish the ribs

1. Preheat one side of the grill to medium.

2. Remove the ribs from the foil and place them on the unheated side of the grill. Cook for 1 hour, turning several times. Every 10 minutes, baste the ribs with the mop sauce to keep them moist.

3. Remove from the grill and let rest for 10 minutes before serving ½ rack per person.

TIP To elevate your dry rub to extraordinary, roast your own cumin seeds before grinding them in a clean spice grinder (or dedicated coffee grinder) or with a mortar and pestle. Place cumin seeds in a small saucepan over medium-low heat and swirl the pan until the seeds are very fragrant.

PER SERVING CALORIES: 428; FAT: 27G; SATURATED FAT: 8G; PROTEIN: 20G; CARBS: 30G; SODIUM: 794; FIBER: 8G; SUGAR: 13G

MAPLE CIDER PORK CHOPS

GLUTEN FREE **PALEO FRIENDLY** QUICK & EASY

SERVES 4 • PREP TIME: 10 MINUTES • COOK TIME: 20 MINUTES

Maple syrup is like any other ingredient; you can purchase excellent quality or not-so-excellent quality. Poorer quality maple syrup is cut with high-fructose corn syrup; good-quality pure maple syrup should come from a reputable source. Use the darkest grade of syrup in this dish, if possible, so the apple cider vinegar perfectly balances the syrup's deep caramel taste.

¼ cup maple syrup

2 tablespoons apple cider vinegar

2 tablespoons chicken broth

2 teaspoons chopped fresh thyme (optional)

4 (5-ounce) bone-in pork loin chops

Sea salt

Freshly ground black pepper

1 tablespoon extra-virgin olive oil

1. In a small nonreactive bowl, stir together the maple syrup, cider vinegar, chicken stock, and thyme (optional).

2. Preheat the oven to 375ºF.

3. Season the pork chops on both sides with sea salt and pepper.

4. Put a large, nonreactive ovenproof skillet over medium-high heat. Add the olive oil. Add the pork chops to the skillet. Sear for 2 minutes on each side.

5. Add the sauce to the skillet and turn the chops to coat.

6. Place the skillet in the preheated oven and bake for about 12 minutes, turning once, or until the pork is just cooked through.

7. Remove from the oven and let the pork rest for 5 minutes. Serve hot.

PER SERVING CALORIES: 448; FAT: 29G; SATURATED FAT: 10G;
PROTEIN: 26G; CARBS: 14G; SODIUM: 106MG; FIBER: 0G; SUGAR: 12G

SPICY SLOPPY JOES

QUICK & EASY

SERVES 4 • PREP TIME: 10 MINUTES • COOK TIME: 20 MINUTES

Sloppy Joes have a murky history with at least three states claiming the invention of this meat sandwich. Ground meat, tomato sauce, onion, and soft buns are the base ingredients, but you can use ground turkey, ground chicken, jalapeños, sweeteners, garlic, and an assortment of spices to make this recipe your own.

---

1 teaspoon extra-virgin olive oil

1 small sweet onion, finely chopped

1 celery stalk, finely chopped

2 teaspoons minced garlic

¾ pound lean ground beef

½ red bell pepper, seeded and chopped

3½ ounces tomato paste

2 tablespoons apple cider vinegar

1 tablespoon molasses

1 teaspoon Dijon mustard

1 teaspoon chili powder

½ teaspoon dried oregano

4 hamburger buns

1. Place a large nonreactive skillet over medium-high heat and add the olive oil. Add the onion, celery, and garlic. Sauté for about 3 minutes, or until translucent.

2. Add the ground beef. Sauté for about 5 minutes, breaking up the meat with a wooden spoon, until the meat is cooked through.

3. Add the bell pepper. Sauté for 2 minutes.

4. Push the meat mixture to the side of the pan and remove any excess oil with a spoon.

5. Add the tomato paste, cider vinegar, molasses, Dijon mustard, chili powder, and oregano, and stir into the meat mixture. Cook for about 10 minutes, stirring occasionally, until very hot and well blended.

6. Serve on the hamburger buns.

 Sloppy Joes benefit from the gentler cooking of a slow cooker. Brown the meat on the stove first with the onion and garlic in a skillet before combining all the ingredients in the cooker. Also increase the liquid in the recipe by adding ½ cup of tomato juice or water.

PER SERVING CALORIES: 342; FAT: 9G; SATURATED FAT: 3G; PROTEIN: 32G; CARBS: 33G; SODIUM: 314MG; FIBER: 3G; SUGAR: 10G

FLANK STEAK WITH CITRUS MARINADE

GLUTEN FREE **PALEO FRIENDLY**

SERVES 4 • PREP TIME: 10 MINUTES, PLUS 2 HOURS MARINATING TIME • COOK TIME: 15 MINUTES

Flank steak is a cut of beef that's usually marinated and grilled to medium-rare. It is incredibly flavorful, but it has tough fibers that need to be cut across the grain after being tenderized. Do not overmarinate the steak in this acidic marinade or the fibers will tighten up instead of loosening.

¼ cup freshly squeezed orange juice

¼ cup freshly squeezed lime juice

1 tablespoon apple cider vinegar

1 teaspoon low-sodium soy sauce

1 tablespoon minced garlic

1 teaspoon grated peeled fresh ginger

1 teaspoon chopped fresh cilantro

1½ pounds flank steak

1. In a small nonreactive bowl, whisk together the orange juice, lime juice, cider vinegar, soy sauce, garlic, ginger, and cilantro.

2. Put the steak in a resealable plastic bag and pour in the marinade. Squeeze out the excess air and seal the bag. Refrigerate the steak to marinate for 2 hours.

3. Preheat the grill to medium-high heat, or an oven to broil.

4. Remove the steak from the marinade and discard the marinade.

5. Grill the steak for about 5 minutes per side for medium, or until the desired doneness. Alternately, broil the steak for about 6 minutes per side for medium, or until the desired doneness.

6. Let the steak rest for 10 minutes before slicing it thinly across the grain. Serve hot.

PER SERVING CALORIES: 346; FAT: 14G; SATURATED FAT: 6G;
PROTEIN: 48G; CARBS: 4G; SODIUM: 144MG; FIBER: 0G; SUGAR: 2G

TRADITIONAL SAUERBRATEN

SERVES 6 • PREP TIME: 20 MINUTES, PLUS 2 DAYS MARINATING TIME • COOK TIME: 3 HOURS, 10 MINUTES

When choosing the beef rump roast for this dish, look for a uniform color that is not too bright, meaning it is not aged. Look for good butchering technique with even smooth cuts that follow the curvature of the muscles, comprehensively trimmed sinew, and enough fat left to keep the meat moist.

---

2 sweet onions, chopped

1 cup apple cider vinegar

½ cup water

2¼ teaspoons sea salt, divided

2¼ teaspoons freshly ground black pepper, divided

1 tablespoon sugar

12 whole cloves

3 dried bay leaves

3 pounds beef rump roast

3 tablespoons all-purpose flour

¼ teaspoon freshly ground black pepper

2 tablespoons extra-virgin olive oil

1 tablespoon cornstarch

1. In a large nonreactive pot, stir together the onions, cider vinegar, water, 2 teaspoons of the sea salt, and the black pepper, sugar, cloves, and bay leaves.

2. Add the roast and turn to coat. Cover the pot and refrigerate. Marinate the beef for 2 days, turning the meat every 8 hours.

3. Remove the beef from the marinade and pat it dry with paper towels. Reserve the marinade.

4. In a small bowl, toss together the flour, remaining ¼ teaspoon of sea salt, and remaining ¼ teaspoon black pepper until well blended. Sprinkle the beef all over with the seasoned flour.

5. Place a large, lidded, nonreactive, ovenproof pot over medium-high heat. Add the olive oil. Add the roast. Brown the meat on all sides for about 10 minutes total. Pour in the reserved marinade. Cover the pot. Reduce the heat to medium-low so the liquid simmers. Simmer the beef for about 3 hours, or until very tender.

6. Transfer the roast to a plate.

7. Increase the heat under the pot to medium. Whisk the cornstarch into the liquid in the pot. Continue to whisk for about 8 minutes, or until the gravy thickens.

8. Pour some of the gravy over the beef and serve hot, and pass the rest of the gravy.

PER SERVING CALORIES: 305; FAT: 9G; SATURATED FAT: 2G; PROTEIN: 44G; CARBS: 11G; SODIUM: 871MG; FIBER: 1G; SUGAR: 4G

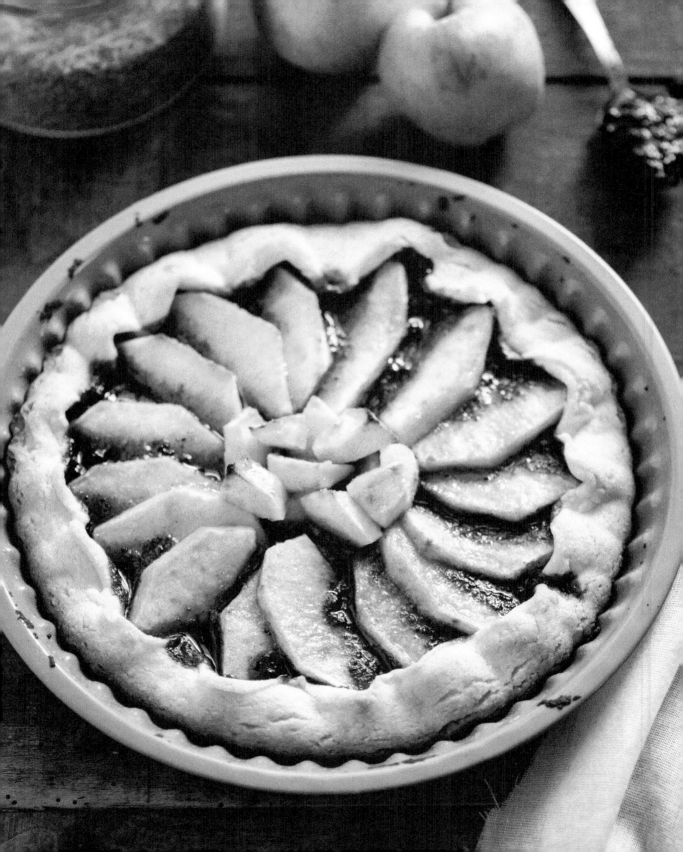

Chapter Eleven

DESSERTS

180   Apple Cider Vinegar Meringues with Raspberries

182   Tangy Panna Cotta with Strawberries

183   Apple Cinnamon Scones

184   Cocoa-Chili Bundt Cake

186   Chocolate-Peanut Butter Cookies

188   Tarte Tatin

190   Apple Cider Vinegar Pie

193   Lemon Pudding Cake

194   Blueberry Cobbler

196   Chocolate Layer Cake

APPLE CIDER VINEGAR MERINGUES WITH RASPBERRIES

GLUTEN FREE **VEGETARIAN**

SERVES 8 • PREP TIME: 30 MINUTES, PLUS 1 HOUR COOLING TIME • COOK TIME: 1 HOUR

The type of meringue used to make these crunchy disks is French meringue. It is simply egg whites beaten with white sugar. It's also the least stable of the meringue choices. If you want to create a truly decadent base for this dessert, add 1 cup of ground nuts, such as almonds or hazelnuts, to the French meringue and bake the meringues as indicated.

6 egg whites, at room temperature

1 tablespoon apple cider vinegar

1 teaspoon vanilla extract

1 teaspoon sea salt

2 cups sugar

2 cups fresh raspberries

1. Preheat the oven to 300°F. Line a baking sheet with parchment paper and set aside.

2. In a large nonreactive bowl, combine the egg whites, cider vinegar, vanilla, and sea salt. Beat the egg whites for about 6 minutes, or until soft peaks form.

3. Continuing beating on low speed, adding the sugar 1 tablespoon at a time, until all the sugar is dissolved and the meringue is thick and glossy, 5 to 7 minutes.

4. With an ice cream scoop or ½-cup measure, drop the meringues onto the prepared sheet about 2 inches apart. You should have 8 meringues. With the back of a spoon, create a well in the center of each meringue.

5. Bake for about 40 minutes, or until the meringues are set.

6. Turn the oven off. Let the meringues cool in the oven with the door closed for 1 hour.

7. Remove the meringues from the oven and cool completely.

8. The meringues will keep for 1 day stored in an airtight container at room temperature.

9. Top with raspberries and serve.

 These sweet, airy meringues can be made with a piping bag fitted with an open star tip to create spectacular nests. Pipe a base circle about 4 inches in diameter. Then create fluted sides, piping around the edge of the base. The meringues will hold their shape as they cook and, once baked, can hold an assortment of fillings, fruit, or mousses.

PER SERVING (1 MERINGUE) CALORIES: 218; FAT: 0G; SATURATED FAT: 0G; PROTEIN: 2G; CARBS: 54G; SODIUM: 259MG; FIBER: 2G; SUGAR: 45G

TANGY PANNA COTTA WITH STRAWBERRIES

GLUTEN FREE VEGETARIAN

SERVES 4 • PREP TIME: 15 MINUTES, PLUS 3 HOURS SETTING TIME • COOK TIME: 10 MINUTES

Gelatin creates the smooth texture of this creamy dessert, and this ingredient needs some special treatment to work effectively. Blooming, or hydrating, the gelatin is essential, and you need to use the gelatin mixture right away or risk ending up with a solid mass you will not want to eat. Do not boil the panna cotta or the gelatin will not set.

---

1 cup whole milk

¼ cup apple cider vinegar

¾ cup heavy (whipping) cream, divided

1 (¼-ounce / 7-gram) packet unflavored gelatin

¼ cup granulated sugar

1 teaspoon vanilla extract

2 cups sliced fresh strawberries

1 tablespoon brown sugar

1. In a small nonreactive bowl, stir together the milk and cider vinegar. Set aside for 10 minutes.

2. Add ¼ cup of the heavy cream to a small saucepan. Sprinkle the gelatin over the cream and let stand for 5 minutes.

3. Place the saucepan over medium-low heat. Cook for about 2 minutes, stirring frequently, or until the gelatin is completely dissolved.

4. Add the remaining ½ cup heavy cream, the granulated sugar, and vanilla to a medium saucepan set over medium heat. Cook for about 5 minutes, stirring, or until the sugar is completely dissolved. Transfer to a large nonreactive measuring cup.

5. Add the cream-gelatin mixture and the milk–cider vinegar mixture to the hot sweetened cream. Stir to combine.

6. Pour the panna cotta into 4 (6-ounce) ramekins. Wrap them in plastic wrap. Refrigerate for about 3 hours, or until set.

7. In a small bowl, stir together the strawberries and brown sugar. Refrigerate for 1 hour.

8. Loosen the panna cotta by running a knife around the inside edges of the ramekins. Invert them onto serving plates.

9. Top with strawberries and serve.

PER SERVING CALORIES: 193; FAT: 9G; SATURATED FAT: 5G; PROTEIN: 4G; CARBS: 24G; SODIUM: 38MG; FIBER: 1G; SUGAR: 21G

APPLE CINNAMON SCONES

QUICK & EASY VEGETARIAN

SERVES 8 • PREP TIME: 15 MINUTES • COOK TIME: 20 MINUTES

You may not think of scones as a dessert, but sometimes all that's needed to end a meal is a slightly sweet treat to accompany a great cup of coffee. The oats and apple create a biscuit-like texture that crumbles in the mouth, while the vinegar adds a tangy finish. If you want a sweeter scone, whisk up a brown sugar glaze to pour over the scones after they cool.

½ cup heavy (whipping) cream

2 tablespoons apple cider vinegar

2⅓ cups all-purpose flour

½ cup rolled oats

1 teaspoon baking powder

½ teaspoon baking soda

1 teaspoon ground cinnamon

1 egg

1 teaspoon vanilla extract

¼ cup maple syrup

1 cup grated apple

1. Preheat the oven to 375°F. Line a baking sheet with parchment paper.

2. In a medium nonreactive bowl, stir together the heavy cream and cider vinegar. Set aside for 10 minutes.

3. In a large nonreactive bowl, whisk together the flour, oats, baking powder, baking soda, and cinnamon. Add the egg, vanilla, maple syrup, and apple. Stir to combine.

4. Add the cream mixture to the flour-egg mixture. Stir until thick and just combined.

5. Turn the batter out onto the prepared baking sheet. Shape it into a round about 1 inch thick.

6. With an oiled pizza cutter or a knife, cut the round into 9 triangles.

7. Bake for about 20 minutes, or until a knife inserted in the center of a scone comes out clean.

8. Cool for 10 minutes on the baking sheet. Separate the scones with a knife.

9. Serve warm.

PER SERVING (1 SCONE) CALORIES: 228; FAT: 4G; SATURATED FAT: 2G; PROTEIN: 6G; CARBS: 42G; SODIUM: 93MG; FIBER: 2G; SUGAR: 8G

COCOA-CHILI BUNDT CAKE

VEGETARIAN

SERVES 10 • PREP TIME: 15 MINUTES • COOK TIME: 35 TO 40 MINUTES

Chocolate and hot chili peppers are a traditional flavor combination that works beautifully in this dense, rich cake. The touch of heat highlights the deep chocolate flavor, creating a unique cake for any event. Sift the dry ingredients the recommended number of times so the chili powder is evenly distributed throughout the batter.

Butter, for the pan

2 cups all-purpose flour, plus more for dusting

¾ cup Dutch-processed cocoa powder

1 teaspoon baking soda

½ teaspoon chili powder

1 cup granulated sugar

¼ teaspoon sea salt

1 cup whole milk

2 eggs

½ cup vegetable oil or melted coconut oil

2 tablespoons apple cider vinegar

1 teaspoon vanilla extract

Confectioners' sugar, for dusting

1. Preheat the oven to 350°F. Lightly butter and flour a 10-inch bundt pan.

2. Into a large nonreactive bowl, sift together the flour, cocoa powder, baking soda, and chili powder at least 3 times. Whisk in the granulated sugar and sea salt.

3. In a medium nonreactive bowl, whisk together the milk, eggs, vegetable oil, cider vinegar, and vanilla.

4. Whisk the milk mixture into the flour mixture until the batter is smooth. Pour the batter into the prepared pan.

5. Bake for 35 to 40 minutes, or until a knife inserted in the center comes out clean.

6. Cool the cake for 10 minutes in the pan and then turn it out onto a wire rack to cool completely.

7. Dust with confectioners' sugar and serve.

PER SERVING CALORIES: 294; FAT: 13G; SATURATED FAT: 3G; PROTEIN: 5G; CARBS: 44G; SODIUM: 196MG; FIBER: 3G; SUGAR: 21G

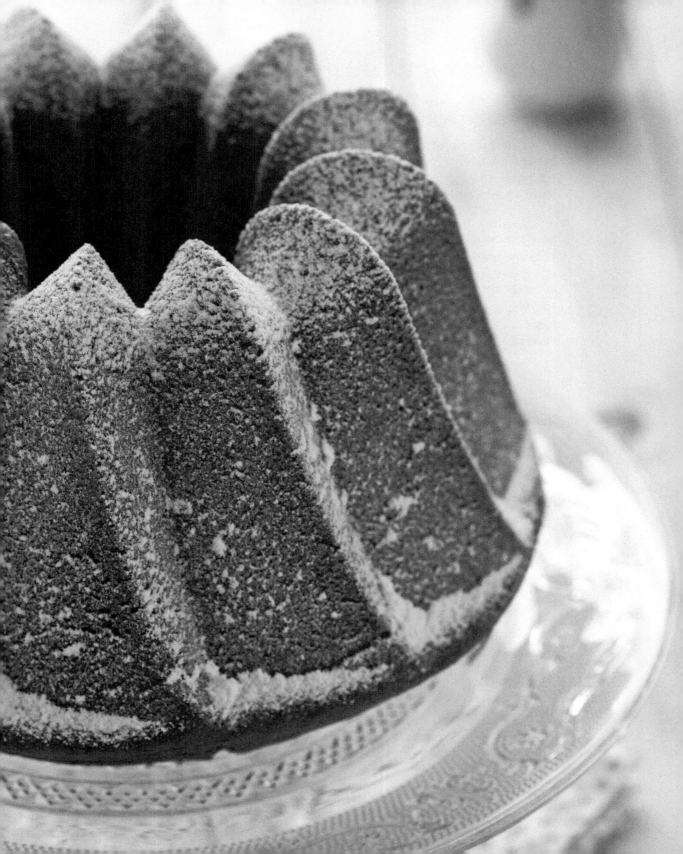

CHOCOLATE-PEANUT BUTTER COOKIES

QUICK & EASY VEGETARIAN

MAKES 24 COOKIES • PREP TIME: 20 MINUTES • COOK TIME: 10 MINUTES

If chocolate is your obsession, you'll find these rich, dense cookies extremely satisfying. The best chocolate for this recipe is dark—the higher the cocoa content, the better. One square of 85 percent dark chocolate is extremely beneficial to your heart's health and doesn't have all the added sugar and fat of sweeter versions.

½ cup dark chocolate chips

¼ cup whole milk

1 cup (2 sticks) unsalted butter, at room temperature

1 cup sugar

2 eggs

1 tablespoon vanilla extract

1 tablespoon apple cider vinegar

2½ cups all-purpose flour

1½ teaspoons baking soda

1 teaspoon baking powder

1 teaspoon sea salt

1 cup peanut butter chips

1. Preheat the oven to 350°F. Line 2 baking sheets with parchment paper.

2. In a medium bowl placed in a pan over, but not touching, gently simmering water, melt the dark chocolate and milk together, whisking constantly. Set aside to cool for 10 minutes.

3. In a large nonreactive bowl, cream together the butter and sugar for about 4 minutes, or until fluffy.

4. Dry the bottom of the bowl with the cooled chocolate. Add the cooled chocolate to the butter-sugar mixture. Beat until well mixed.

5. Beat in the eggs, one at a time, scraping the bowl after each addition.

6. Beat in the vanilla and cider vinegar, scraping the sides of the bowl as needed.

7. In a medium bowl, whisk together the flour, baking soda, baking powder, and sea salt.

8. Stir the flour mixture into the chocolate mixture until blended.

9. Stir in the peanut butter chips.

10. By tablespoons, scoop the dough onto the prepared pans about 1 inch apart and press down lightly to flatten.

11. Bake for about 10 minutes, or until firm on the edges.

12. Cool for 3 minutes on the baking sheets. Transfer the cookies to a wire rack to cool completely.

13. Store the cookies in a sealed container for up to 1 week at room temperature or in the refrigerator, or in the freezer for 2 months.

TIP Omit the peanut butter chips and make a peanut butter cream instead, to create especially irresistible sandwich cookies for a birthday party or special event. Just beat ¾ cup confectioners' sugar, ½ cup smooth peanut butter, ½ teaspoon melted butter, and 1 teaspoon vanilla until smooth. You can make the cookies ahead and fill them on the day needed, to save time.

PER SERVING (1 COOKIE) CALORIES: 221; FAT: 12G; SATURATED FAT: 8G; PROTEIN: 2G; CARBS: 27G; SODIUM: 248MG; FIBER: 0G; SUGAR: 16G

TARTE TATIN

VEGETARIAN

SERVES 8 • PREP TIME: 20 MINUTES • COOK TIME: 1 HOUR

If you're like most cooks, you probably use any type of apple you have on hand when needed for a recipe. Luckily all apples tend to work well in most applications, but some varieties are better than others for desserts like this scrumptious tart. Texture is important when choosing apples for Tarte Tatin because you want them to hold their shape and not get mushy. Try Courtland, Honeycrisp, or Pink Lady for this rustic tart, or a combination.

---

1 cup sugar

¼ cup water

1 sheet puff pastry, thawed

6 Honeycrisp apples, peeled, cored, and cut into eighths

½ cup blackberry preserves

2 tablespoons apple cider vinegar

3 tablespoons cold butter

Flour, for dusting

1. Preheat the oven to 400°F.

2. In a 9-inch, nonreactive ovenproof skillet set over medium heat, combine the sugar and water, stirring to dissolve the sugar. Swirl the sugar water over the heat for about 5 minutes, or until it is caramelized and a deep amber color. Remove the skillet from the heat.

3. Carefully stir in the preserves, cider vinegar, and butter because the hot caramel can spatter.

4. Carefully arrange the apple slices in a single, slightly overlapping layer in the skillet, taking care with the hot caramel.

5. Place the skillet back over medium heat. Cook for 10 minutes. Remove the skillet from the heat and set aside.

6. Lightly dust a clean work surface with flour. Roll the puff pastry into an 11-inch square. Prick the surface all over with a fork.

7. Place the puff pastry over the apples. Trim the edges so the pastry is roughly round. Tuck the edges into the skillet.

8. Place the skillet in the preheated oven and bake for 30 minutes. Remove from the oven and cool for 5 minutes.

9. Invert a large plate over the top of the skillet. Wearing oven mitts, hold the plate and skillet together and carefully flip them over so the plate is on the bottom. Lift off the skillet slowly. If any apple slices stick to the pan, slide them off onto the tart with a spatula.

10. Serve warm.

 Making puff pastry used to be an arduous task that required a deft hand, lots of time, and cool, dry weather. Now you can pick up a package of ready-made product in the freezer and refrigerated sections of the grocery store. This recipe can be made with pie crust pastry as well, if you have some on hand.

PER SERVING CALORIES: 254; FAT: 6G; SATURATED FAT: 4G; PROTEIN: 1G; CARBS: 48G; SODIUM: 85MG; FIBER: 4G; SUGAR: 42G

APPLE CIDER VINEGAR PIE

VEGETARIAN

SERVES 8 • PREP TIME: 30 MINUTES, PLUS 2 HOURS CHILLING TIME • COOK TIME: 1 HOUR

Vinegar pie is an extremely old recipe traditionally served in the winter when fresh fruit was not available for baking. References to this dish can be found in the popular Laura Ingalls Wilder book Little House in the Big Woods. *Do not let the amount of water in this filling scare you; the final result will be creamy and light.*

For the crust

1 cup plus 2 tablespoons all-purpose flour

2 teaspoons sugar

¼ teaspoon sea salt

½ cup (1 stick) butter, chilled and cut into ½-inch cubes

4 to 5 tablespoons ice water

1 teaspoon apple cider vinegar

For the filling

2 eggs

1 cup sugar, divided

1 tablespoon all-purpose flour

1 cup cold water

2 tablespoons apple cider vinegar

To make the crust

1. In a food processor, combine the flour, sugar, and sea salt. Pulse a few times to combine. Add the cold butter. Pulse until the butter pieces are pea size. (You can also make the crust in a large bowl. Stir together the flour, sugar, and sea salt until combined, and then cut the cold butter into the flour mixture with two knives or a pastry blender until the mixture is a coarse meal with pea-size butter bits.)

2. In a small nonreactive bowl, stir together the water and cider vinegar. Add to the food processor and pulse until the dough starts to hold together. (Or add to the dry pastry mixture 1 tablespoon at a time until the dough starts to hold together.)

3. Turn the dough out onto a piece of plastic wrap. Wrap it tightly, shaping it so it holds together as a ball. Refrigerate for 2 hours.

4. Preheat the oven to 400°F.

5. Lightly flour a clean work surface. Unwrap the dough, place it on the surface, and using a rolling pin, roll into a 12-inch round.

6. Fit the dough into a 10-inch pie plate. Trim the excess, leaving a ½-inch overhang. Fold the overhang over to form a rim and crimp the edges.

7. Line the pie shell with aluminum foil. Fill with dried beans or pie weights.

8. Place the pie shell in the middle of the preheated oven and bake for about 20 minutes, or until the edge is pale golden and sides are set. Remove from the oven, remove the pie weights, and set aside.

9. Reduce the oven temperature to 350°F.

To make the filling

1. In a medium bowl, whisk together the eggs and ¼ cup of the sugar until well blended.

2. In a large nonreactive saucepan, whisk together the flour and remaining ¾ cup sugar. Add the water and cider vinegar to the flour mixture. Whisk to combine.

3. Place the pan over medium-high heat. Bring the mixture to a boil. Whisk for about 3 minutes, or until the sugar is completely dissolved.

4. Whisk in the egg mixture. Reduce the heat to low. Cook the filling for about 15 minutes, stirring constantly, until it reaches 175°F on a candy thermometer and coats the back of a spoon.

5. Pour the filling into the pie shell. Cover the edge of the pie crust with narrow pieces of foil to keep it from overbrowning.

6. Bake for about 20 minutes, or until the filling is set and the tip of a sharp knife inserted into the filling midway between the edge and the center comes out clean.

7. Cool completely and serve.

PER SERVING CALORIES: 279; FAT: 13G; SATURATED FAT: 7G;
PROTEIN: 3G; CARBS: 39G; SODIUM: 173MG; FIBER: 0G; SUGAR: 26G

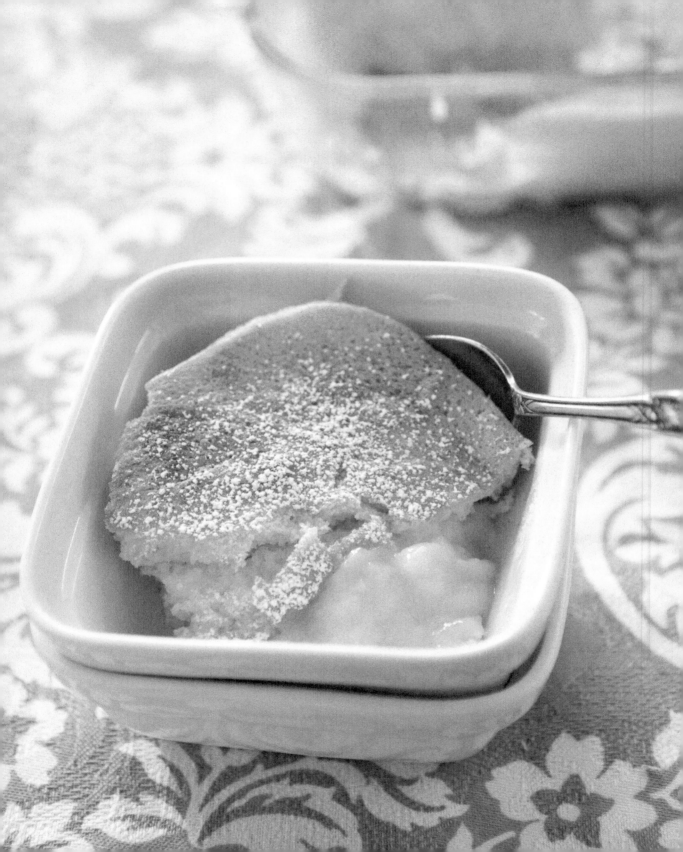

LEMON PUDDING CAKE

VEGETARIAN

SERVES 6 • PREP TIME: 30 MINUTES • COOK TIME: 35 MINUTES

Lemon desserts are a favorite flavor worldwide. The intense lemon flavor in this pudding cake is, in part, due to the essential oils in the lemon zest.

---

2 tablespoons salted butter, melted, plus more for the pan

1 cup whole milk

¼ cup apple cider vinegar

3 eggs, separated, at room temperature

¾ cup sugar

½ cup all-purpose flour

Pinch sea salt

Zest of 1 lemon

Juice of 1 lemon

1. Preheat the oven to 350°F. Lightly butter an 8-by-8-inch baking pan.

2. In a small nonreactive bowl, stir together the milk and cider vinegar. Set aside for 10 minutes.

3. In a large nonreactive bowl, beat together the egg yolks and sugar until pale yellow and fluffy.

4. Add the flour and sea salt to the yolk mixture. Beat to combine, scraping down the sides of the bowl at least once.

5. Add the milk–cider vinegar mixture, lemon zest, lemon juice, and melted butter. Whisk the batter until well mixed.

6. In another large bowl, beat the egg whites for about 4 minutes, or until soft peaks form. Gently fold the egg whites into the batter until just blended.

7. Transfer the batter to the prepared pan and set the pan inside a large baking dish. Place the baking dish in the center of the preheated oven. Carefully pour hot water into the large baking dish until it comes up about 1 inch on the sides of the smaller baking pan.

8. Bake for about 35 minutes, or until the top is puffed and golden.

9. Remove the cake pan from the water bath. Cool on a rack for 30 minutes.

 TIP The batter for this cake separates into a light spongy top and rich pudding bottom while it cooks. The water bath ensures even cooking with lots of moisture, so do not skip this step in the process.

PER SERVING CALORIES: 224; FAT: 7G; SATURATED FAT: 4G;
PROTEIN: 5G; CARBS: 35G; SODIUM: 102MG; FIBER: 0G; SUGAR: 27G

BLUEBERRY COBBLER

VEGETARIAN

SERVES 8 • PREP TIME: 20 MINUTES • COOK TIME: 35 MINUTES

Cobbler recipes are incredibly forgiving to ingredient substitutions. The milk in this recipe can be swapped with almond milk and the butter replaced by chilled coconut oil to make it vegan. Also, the cobbler topping can be made with almond flour instead of all-purpose flour if you need a gluten-free dessert. Do not be afraid to experiment with the ingredients of this deeply satisfying old-fashioned dessert.

For the filling
6 cups fresh blueberries
½ cup sugar
1½ tablespoons cornstarch
1 teaspoon vanilla extract

For the cobbler topping
½ cup whole milk
¼ cup apple cider vinegar
1½ cups all-purpose flour
¼ cup sugar
1 teaspoon baking powder
1 teaspoon ground ginger
¼ teaspoon ground nutmeg
Pinch sea salt
4 tablespoons cold butter, cut into ½-inch cubes

To make the filling

1. In a large bowl, toss together the blueberries, sugar, cornstarch, and vanilla.
2. Transfer to an 8-by-8-inch baking dish. Set aside.

To make the cobbler topping

1. Preheat the oven to 400°F.
2. In a small nonreactive bowl, stir together the milk and cider vinegar. Set aside for 10 minutes.
3. In a large nonreactive bowl, whisk together the flour, sugar, baking powder, ginger, nutmeg, and sea salt.
4. Add the butter. Using 2 knives or a pastry blender, cut the butter into the flour mixture until the mixture resembles coarse crumbs.
5. Add the milk mixture in a thin stream to the flour-butter crumbs, tossing the ingredients with a fork until a sticky dough forms.

6. With a tablespoon, scoop the dough over the blueberries, spacing the mounds as evenly as possible and leaving spaces here and there for steam to escape.

7. Place the baking dish on a baking pan (to catch blueberry filling drips) and bake for about 35 minutes, or until the cobbler topping is golden brown and the blueberries are bubbly.

8. Serve warm.

 Cobbler is a versatile dessert that is wonderful with any fruit or combination of fruit. Strawberries, peaches, apples, rhubarb, plums, pears, and cherries all stand in for blueberries. Some fruit is juicier than others, so increase the cornstarch just a bit if you have very ripe peaches or cherries.

PER SERVING CALORIES: 288; FAT: 7G; SATURATED FAT: 4G;
PROTEIN: 4G; CARBS: 55G; SODIUM: 69MG; FIBER: 3G; SUGAR: 30G

CHOCOLATE LAYER CAKE

VEGETARIAN

SERVES 12 TO 16 • PREP TIME: 45 MINUTES, PLUS 1 HOUR, 30 MINUTES CHILLING TIME • COOK TIME: 30 MINUTES

Chocolate has many of the same benefits of dark leafy vegetables, like antioxidants and flavonoids, which are extremely beneficial for the heart. Dark chocolate has been proven to lower cholesterol and blood pressure by impressive amounts. It's important to taste the chocolate you use to gauge the impact its texture and flavor will have on the finished product. Some lower quality chocolate has a waxy mouthfeel and performs poorly when melted. Choose a chocolate that is reputed to be an excellent baking chocolate.

For the cake

Butter, for the cake pans

1½ cups all-purpose flour, plus more for dusting

1 cup granulated sugar

½ cup Dutch-processed cocoa powder

1 teaspoon baking soda

1 teaspoon sea salt

⅓ cup vegetable oil or melted coconut oil

¼ cup whole milk

1½ tablespoons apple cider vinegar

1 cup semi-sweet mini chocolate chips

For the frosting

5 ounces semi-sweet chocolate

3 ounces unsweetened chocolate

½ cup (1 stick) unsalted butter

½ cup heavy (whipping) cream

1½ cups confectioners' sugar

2 teaspoons vanilla extract

To make the cake

1. Preheat the oven to 350°F. Lightly butter and dust 2 (6-inch) cake pans.

2. In a large nonreactive bowl, stir together the flour, granulated sugar, cocoa powder, baking soda, and sea salt.

3. In a medium nonreactive bowl, whisk together the vegetable oil, milk, and cider vinegar.

4. Add the oil mixture to the flour mixture and stir until just combined. Do not overmix.

5. Stir in the chocolate chips.

6. Pour the batter, evenly divided, into the prepared pans. Bake for 25 to 30 minutes, or until a knife inserted in the center comes out clean.

7. Cool the cakes in the pans for 10 minutes. Run a knife around the edges of the cakes and turn them out onto wire racks to cool completely.

8. Wrap the cooled cakes in plastic wrap and refrigerate for about 1 hour 30 minutes, or until completely chilled.

To make the frosting

1. In a medium nonreactive bowl placed in a pan over but not touching gently simmering water, melt together the semi-sweet chocolate, unsweetened chocolate, and butter, whisking constantly.

2. Remove the melted chocolate from the heat and whisk in the heavy cream.

3. Add the confectioners' sugar in four batches, whisking well after each addition, until all the sugar is well incorporated.

4. Add the vanilla, whisking until the icing is very smooth and fluffy.

To assemble the cake

1. Once the cakes are chilled, remove them from the refrigerator. Place them right-side up on a work surface. With a sharp serrated knife, level the tops.

2. Place one cake on a plate. Spread one-fourth of the frosting on the top.

3. Top with the second cake, pressing gently to adhere. Spread one-fourth of the frosting on the top.

4. Frost the sides of the cake with the remaining half of the chocolate frosting. Cut and serve.

PER SERVING CALORIES: 372; FAT: 20G; SATURATED FAT: 10G; PROTEIN: 4G; CARBS: 48G; SODIUM: 280MG; FIBER: 2G; SUGAR: 34G

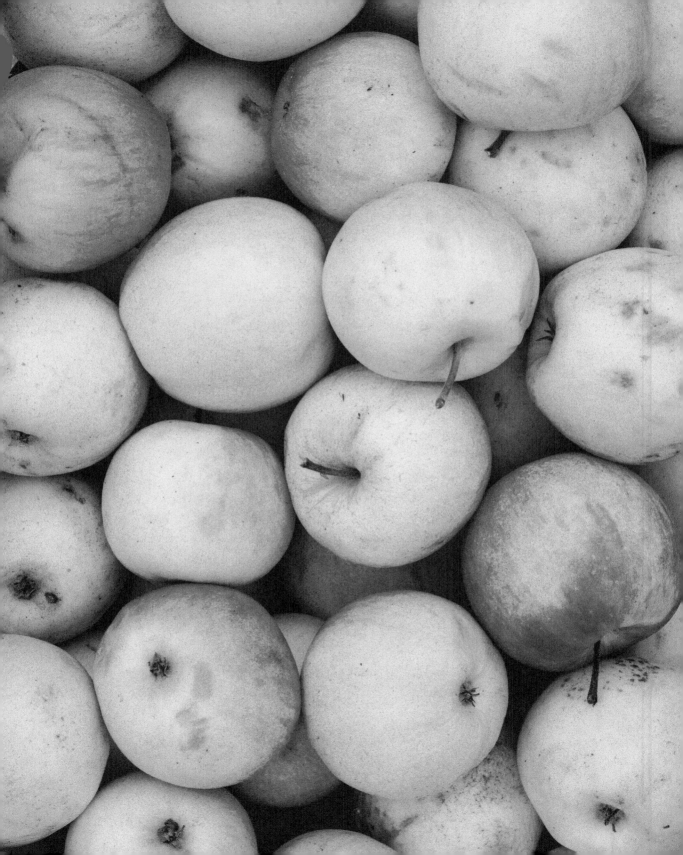

CONVERSION TABLES

VOLUME EQUIVALENTS (LIQUID)

US STANDARD	US STANDARD (OUNCES)	METRIC (APPROXIMATE)
2 tablespoons	1 fl. oz.	30 mL
¼ cup	2 fl. oz.	60 mL
½ cup	4 fl. oz.	120 mL
1 cup	8 fl. oz.	240 mL
1½ cups	12 fl. oz.	355 mL
2 cups or 1 pint	16 fl. oz.	475 mL
4 cups or 1 quart	32 fl. oz.	1 L
1 gallon	128 fl. oz.	4 L

VOLUME EQUIVALENTS (DRY)

US STANDARD	METRIC (APPROXIMATE)
⅛ teaspoon	0.5 mL
¼ teaspoon	1 mL
½ teaspoon	2 mL
¾ teaspoon	4 mL
1 teaspoon	5 mL
1 tablespoon	15 mL
¼ cup	59 mL
⅓ cup	79 mL
½ cup	118 mL
⅔ cup	156 mL
¾ cup	177 mL
1 cup	235 mL
2 cups or 1 pint	475 mL
3 cups	700 mL
4 cups or 1 quart	1 L

OVEN TEMPERATURES

FAHRENHEIT (F)	CELSIUS (C) (APPROXIMATE)
250°F	120°C
300°F	150°C
325°F	165°C
350°F	180°C
375°F	190°C
400°F	200°C
425°F	220°C
450°F	230°C

WEIGHT EQUIVALENTS

US STANDARD	METRIC (APPROXIMATE)
½ ounce	15 g
1 ounce	30 g
2 ounces	60 g
4 ounces	115 g
8 ounces	225 g
12 ounces	340 g
16 ounces or 1 pound	455 g

THE DIRTY DOZEN
& THE CLEAN FIFTEEN

A nonprofit environmental watchdog organization called Environmental Working Group (EWG) looks at data supplied by the US Department of Agriculture (USDA) and the Food and Drug Administration (FDA) about pesticide residues. Each year it compiles a list of the best and worst pesticide loads found in commercial crops. You can use these lists to decide which fruits and vegetables to buy organic to minimize your exposure to pesticides and which produce is considered safe enough to buy conventionally. This does not mean they are pesticide-free, though, so wash these fruits and vegetables thoroughly.

These lists change every year, so make sure you look up the most recent one before you fill your shopping cart. You'll find the most recent lists as well as a guide to pesticides in produce at EWG.org/FoodNews.

2015 Dirty Dozen

Apples	Peaches	*In addition to the Dirty Dozen, the EWG added two types of produce contaminated with highly toxic organo-phosphate insecticides:*
Celery	Potatoes	
Cherry tomatoes	Snap peas (imported)	
Cucumbers	Spinach	
Grapes	Strawberries	Kale/Collard greens
Nectarines (imported)	Sweet bell peppers	Hot peppers

2015 Clean Fifteen

Asparagus	Eggplants	Papayas
Avocados	Grapefruits	Pineapples
Cabbage	Kiwis	Sweet corn
Cantaloupes (domestic)	Mangoes	Sweet peas (frozen)
Cauliflower	Onions	Sweet potatoes

RESOURCES

**For essential oils,
carrier oils, and oil blends:**

Young Living
www.youngliving.com

**For glassware, containers,
and bottles:**

Life Science Products & Publishing
www.discoverlsp.com

**For herbs, spices, and teas
to use in your home remedies:**

Spicely
www.spicely.com

**For raw, unfiltered,
commercial apple cider vinegar:**

Bragg Live Foods
www.bragg.com

Spectrum
www.spectrumorganics.com

**For teas, herbs, and florals
to use in your home remedies:**

Mountain Rose Herbs
www.mountainroseherbs.com

REFERENCES

Atwood, Rebecca. *The New Whole Foods Encyclopedia*. New York: Penguin Books, 2010.

Budak, Nilgün H., et al. "Functional Properties of Vinegar." *Journal of Food Science* 74, no. 5 (May 2014). R757–R764. doi:10.1111/1750-3841.12434.

Entani, E., M. Asai, S. Tsujihata, Y. Tsukamoto, and M. Ohta. "Antibacterial Action of Vinegar Against Food-Borne Pathogenic Bacteria Including *Escherichia Coli* O157:H7." *Journal of Food Protection* 61, no. 8 (August 1998): 953–9. Accessed July 7, 2015. National Center for Biotechnology Information. www.ncbi.nlm.nih.gov/pubmed/9713753.

Fournie, Daniel A. "Second Punic War: Hannibal's War in Italy." HistoryNet. Accessed July 5, 2015. www.historynet.com/second-punic-war-hannibals-war-in-italy.htm

Hellmiss, Margot. *Natural Healing with Apple Cider Vinegar*. New York: Sterling Publishing, 1998.

Jian Chen, and Yang Zhu. *Solid State Fermentation for Foods and Beverages*. Boca Raton, FL: CRC Press, 2014.

Johnston, Carol S., and Gaas, Cindy A. "Vinegar: Medicinal Uses and Antiglycemic Effect." *Medscape General Medicine* 8, no. 2 (2006): 6. Published online May 2006. www.ncbi.nlm.nih.gov/pmc/articles/PMC1785201/.

Jones, Bridget. *Vinegar & Oil*. London: Anness Publishing, 2010.

Lorenzi, Rossella. "How Cleopatra Won Her Bet." Discovery News. November 27, 2012. news.discovery.com/history/ancient-egypt/cleopatra-pearl-cocktail.htm.

McLean, Matilda. "The Acid Test for Arthritis." The Telegraph. August 6, 2007. www.telegraph.co.uk/news/health/3350714/The-acid-test-for-arthritis.html.

Mercola, Joseph MD. "What the Research Really Says About Apple Cider Vinegar." Mercola.com. June 2, 2009. Articles.mercola.com/sites/articles/archive/2009/06/02/apple-cider-vinegar-hype.aspx.

Oster, Maggie. *Herbal Vinegar*. Pownal, VT: Storey Communications, 1994.

Shinohara, K., Y. Ohashi, K. Kawasumi, A. Terada, and T. Fujisawa. "Effect of Apple Intake on Fecal Microbiota and Metabolites in Humans." *Anaerobe* 16, no. 5 (October 2010): 510–5. doi: 10.1016/j.anaerobe.2010.03.005. Epub March 19, 2010. National Center for Biotechnology Information. Accessed July 6, 2015. www.ncbi.nlm.nih.gov/pubmed/20304079.

Shishehbor, F., A. Mansoori, A. R. Sarkaki, M. T. Jalali, and S. M. Latifi. "Antibacterial Action of Vinegar Against Food-Borne Pathogenic Bacteria Including *Escherichia coli* O157:H7." *Pakistan Journal of Biological Sciences* 11, no. 23 (2008): 2634–38. doi:10.3923/pjbs.2008.2634.2638. National Center for Biotechnology Information. Accessed July 6, 2015. www.ncbi.nlm.nih.gov/pubmed/19630216.

REMEDY & RECIPE INDEX

A

Activated Charcoal and Clay Facial Pack, 45
Allium Ear Dropper, 77
Almond-Berry Smoothie, 96
Aloe Vera-Turmeric Gel Facial, 54
Aloe-Lemon Shooter, 79
Antifungal Tea Tree Nail Soak, 51
Apple Cider Vinegar Meringues with Raspberries, 180–181
Apple Cider Vinegar Pie, 190–191
Apple Cinnamon Scones, 183
Apple Pie Drink, 92
Applesauce and Papaya Purée Peel, 55
Asian Asparagus Salad, 154
Avocado-Herb Smoothie, 104

B

Bacon and Cheddar Breakfast Scones, 113
Banana-Berry Smoothie, 105
Basic Apple Cider Vinegar Facial Toner, 44
Bavarian Braised Red Cabbage, 135
Berry Vinaigrette, 126
Black Salve, 75
Blueberry Cobbler, 194–195
Blueberry Muffins, 110
Bone Broth Sipper, 84
Bright Carrot Smoothie, 103

C

Castor Oil and Witch Hazel Makeup Remover, 48
Chamomile Conditioning Rinse, 60
Cherry-Apple Cider Nectar, 66
Chicken-Broccoli Soup, 141
Chicken Pot Pie, 165–166

Chili Dry Rub Pork Ribs, 172–173
Chinese Chicken Lettuce Wraps, 169
Chocolate Layer Cake, 196–197
Chocolate Mineral Smoothie, 81
Chocolate-Peanut Butter Cookies, 186–187
Cinnamon Apple Breakfast Cake, 111
Citrus Cypress Spray, 58
Citrus Joint Juice, 67
Citrus Refresher, 91
Cocoa-Chili Bundt Cake, 184
Cracked Heel Salve with Rice Cream, 51
Creamy Mashed Potatoes, 134
Creamy Peach Smoothie, 106
Creamy Scrambled Eggs, 119
Cucumber-Lemon Cleanser, 63
Curried Root Vegetable Soup, 142

D

Dark Chocolate Pancakes, 115
Double Almond Muffins, 114

E

Eggs Poached in Ratatouille, 118
Elderberry Shrub, 70
Essential Earache Rub, 76
Exfoliating Lemon-Sugar Scalp Scrub, 47

F

Fennel Tea, 83
Fennel-Jicama Salad, 152
Fire Cider, 69
Flaky Biscuit and Egg Sandwiches, 120–121
Flank Steak with Citrus Marinade, 176
Four Thieves Vinegar, 71

G

Garlic Dill Pickles, 133
Gazpacho Smoothie, 102
Ginger Switchel, 82
Golden French Toast, 116
Greek Couscous Salad, 149
Green Goddess Dressing, 129
Grilled Vegetable Pasta Salad, 150

H

Hair-Shining Tea and Sea Spray, 61
Herb-Flower Vinegar, 130
Herb-Marinated Halibut, 163
Homemade Apple Cider Vinegar, 38
Homemade Beef Stock, 138
Homemade Chicken Stock, 139
Honey Tomato Chicken Drumsticks, 168
Honey-Lemon Tea, 93
Hot and Sour Soup, 140

I

Irish Bannock, 112

L

Lavender Scalp Toner, 62
Lavender-Coconut Hair Mask, 61
Lavender-Oatmeal Soak, 57
Lemon Pudding Cake, 193
Lemon-Lavender Hand Spray, 53
Licorice Root Gargle, 85
Lime and Mint Salt Scrub, 50
Lime-Cider Soda, 94
Linguine Carbonara, 170
Lip-Lightening Paste, 55

M

Magnesium Massage Oil, 59
Mango Skin Slougher, 49
Mango-Ginger Smoothie, 97
Maple Cider Pork Chops, 174
Maple Salmon Packets with Asian
    Vegetables, 167
Mustard Chicken Salad, 146

N

Nettle and Tea Tree Rinse, 46

O

Oktoberfest Stew, 145
Orange-Coconut Constipation
    Chews, 73

P

Parched Skin Peppermint
    Spray, 56
PB and J Smoothie, 99
Pear Green Smoothie, 101
Peppermint, Ginger, and Fennel
    Sipper, 78

Plantain Poultice, 74
Potato Salad with Hot Bacon
    Dressing, 151
Pre-Mani Nail Soak, 52
Psyllium Solution, 72
Pumpkin Pie Enzyme Mask, 45

R

Raspberry Lemonade, 90
Roasted Maple Celeriac, 131
Roasted Tomato Soup, 144
Rosemary–Epsom Salts Soak, 59
Rosewater and Sea Salt Body
    Spray, 49

S

Scallops with Bacon Cream
    Sauce, 162
Spiced Carrot Salad, 147
Spicy Sloppy Joes, 175
Sun-Dried Tomato Vinaigrette, 128
Sweet and Spicy Barbecue
    Sauce, 125

T

Tahini Curry Noodle Bowl,
    158–159
Tangy Panna Cotta with
    Strawberries, 182
Tarte Tatin, 188–189
Tender Tummy Rub, 73
Tomato Ketchup, 124
Traditional Sauerbraten, 177
Tropical Cider Smoothie, 98

V

Vinegar Vapor for Stuffy
    Sinuses, 68

W

Warm Mint Compress, 80
Watermelon-Tomato Salad, 155
Wheat Berry-Stuffed
    Tomatoes, 161
Wild Rice Bowl, 160

INDEX

A

Acetic acid, 22
Acetic acid bacteria (AAB), 22–23
Acne, 25, 26
  Activated Charcoal and Clay
    Facial Pack, 45
  Basic Apple Cider Vinegar
    Facial Toner, 44
  Pumpkin Pie Enzyme Mask, 45
Activated charcoal
  Activated Charcoal and Clay
    Facial Pack, 45
  Black Salve, 75
Allergies, 26
  apple cider vinegar and, 24
Allium Ear Dropper, 77
Allspice
  Tomato Ketchup, 124
Almond-Berry Smoothie, 96
Almond extract
  Double Almond Muffins, 114
Almond milk
  Almond-Berry Smoothie, 96
  Chocolate Mineral Smoothie, 81
  Mango-Ginger Smoothie, 97
  PB and J Smoothie, 99
Almonds
  Mustard Chicken Salad, 146
  Spiced Carrot Salad, 147
Aloe vera gel
  Aloe-Lemon Shooter, 79
  Aloe Vera-Turmeric Gel
    Facial, 54
  Hair-Shining Tea and Sea
    Spray, 61
  Parched Skin Peppermint
    Spray, 56
  Rosewater and Sea Salt Body
    Spray, 49
Antifungal Tea Tree Nail Soak, 51

Apple cider vinegar
  amount consumed, 29
  core ingredients in, 32–33
  defined, 14
  evaluating and bottling, 34
  in food, 19
  frequently asked questions
    about, 28–29
  in history and culture, 18–19
  homemade, 31–38
  making, 14
  in medicine, 18
  nutrition and, 8
  organic, 29, 32
  pH value of, 28
  precautions with, 24
  as probiotic, 29
  raw versus pasteurized, 15–16
  reasons for making your own, 16
  science on, 22–23
  storage of, 28
  unfiltered versus filtered, 15
  uses of, 8–9, 14, 21, 22
  versatility of, 28
Apple Cider Vinegar Meringues
    with Raspberries, 180–181
Apple Cider Vinegar Pie, 190–191
Apple Cinnamon Scones, 183
Apple juice
  Apple Pie Drink, 92
  Avocado-Herb Smoothie, 104
  Bright Carrot Smoothie, 103
  Creamy Peach Smoothie, 106
  Pear Green Smoothie, 101
Apples, 32
  Apple Cinnamon Scones, 183
  Cinnamon Apple Breakfast
    Cake, 111
  Curried Root Vegetable
    Soup, 142
  Fennel-Jicama Salad, 152

  Mustard Chicken Salad, 146
  Tarte Tatin, 188–189
Applesauce and Papaya Purée
    Peel, 55
Argan oil
  Exfoliating Lemon-Sugar Scalp
    Scrub, 47
Arthritis, 25
  Cherry-Apple Cider Nectar, 66
  Citrus Joint Juice, 67
Arugula
  Fennel-Jicama Salad, 152
Asian Asparagus Salad, 154
Asparagus
  Asian Asparagus Salad, 154
  Grilled Vegetable Pasta
    Salad, 150
Athlete's foot, 26
Avocado
  Avocado-Herb Smoothie, 104
  Chocolate Mineral Smoothie, 81
  Green Goddess Dressing, 129
Avocado oil
  Lime and Mint Salt Scrub, 50
  Parched Skin Peppermint
    Spray, 56
  Tender Tummy Rub, 73

B

Bacon
  Bacon and Cheddar Breakfast
    Scones, 113
  Linguine Carbonara, 170
  Potato Salad with Hot Bacon
    Dressing, 151
  Scallops with Bacon Cream
    Sauce, 162
Baking soda
  Antifungal Tea Tree Nail Soak, 51
  Lavender-Oatmeal Soak, 57
Bald spots, 26

Bananas
  Almond-Berry Smoothie, 96
  Banana-Berry Smoothie, 105
  Chocolate Mineral Smoothie, 81
  Creamy Peach Smoothie, 106
  Mango-Ginger Smoothie, 97
  PB and J Smoothie, 99
  Tropical Cider Smoothie, 98
Basic Apple Cider Vinegar Facial
    Toner, 44
Basil
  Berry Vinaigrette, 126
  Eggs Poached in Ratatouille, 118
  Fennel-Jicama Salad, 152
  Greek Couscous Salad, 149
  Green Goddess Dressing, 129
  Grilled Vegetable Pasta
    Salad, 150
  Herb-Marinated Halibut, 163
  Linguine Carbonara, 170
  Roasted Tomato Soup, 144
  Sun-Dried Tomato
    Vinaigrette, 128
  Wheat Berry-Stuffed
    Tomatoes, 161
Bay leaves
  Homemade Beef Stock, 138
  Homemade Chicken Stock, 139
  Traditional Sauerbraten, 177
Bean sprouts
  Chinese Chicken Lettuce
    Wraps, 169
  Maple Salmon Packets with
    Asian Vegetables, 167
Beef
  Flank Steak with Citrus
    Marinade, 176
  Traditional Sauerbraten, 177
Beef bones
  Homemade Beef Stock, 138
Beer
  Oktoberfest Stew, 145
Beeswax
  Black Salve, 75
Bentonite clay
  Activated Charcoal and Clay
    Facial Pack, 45
  Black Salve, 75

Berry Vinaigrette, 126
Black Salve, 75
Blood sugar regulation, 26
Blueberries
  Banana-Berry Smoothie, 105
  Blueberry Cobbler, 194–195
  Blueberry Muffin, 110
Bok choy
  Hot and Sour Soup, 140
  Maple Salmon Packets with
    Asian Vegetables, 167
Bone Broth Sipper, 84
Boston lettuce
  Chinese Chicken Lettuce
    Wraps, 169
Bavarian Braised Red Cabbage, 135
Breakfast
  Bacon and Cheddar Breakfast
    Scones, 113
  Blueberry Muffins, 110
  Cinnamon Apple Breakfast
    Cake, 111
  Creamy Scrambled Eggs, 119
  Dark Chocolate Pancakes, 115
  Double Almond Muffins, 114
  Eggs Poached in Ratatouille, 118
  Flaky Biscuit and Egg
    Sandwiches, 120–121
  Golden French Toast, 116
  Irish Bannock, 112
Brewing container, 33
Bright Carrot Smoothie, 103
Broccoli slaw
  Chicken-Broccoli Soup, 141
Brown sugar
  Exfoliating Lemon-Sugar Scalp
    Scrub, 47
Burns
  apple cider vinegar and, 24

C

Cabbage. See Green cabbage;
    Napa cabbage; Red cabbage
Calendula flowers
  Hair-Shining Tea and Sea
    Spray, 61
  Rosemary-Epsom Salts Soak, 59
Candida overgrowth, 26

Caraway seeds
  Oktoberfest Stew, 145
Carrier oil
  Lime and Mint Salt Scrub, 50
Carrots
  Bright Carrot Smoothie, 103
  Chicken Pot Pie, 165–166
  Chinese Chicken Lettuce
    Wraps, 169
  Curried Root Vegetable
    Soup, 142
  Homemade Beef Stock, 138
  Homemade Chicken Stock, 139
  Maple Salmon Packets with
    Asian Vegetables, 167
  Spiced Carrot Salad, 147
  Tahini Curry Noodle Bowl,
    158–159
  Wild Rice Bowl, 160
Carrot seed essential oil
  Castor Oil and Witch Hazel
    Makeup Remover, 48
  Pre-Mani Nail Soak, 52
Cashews
  Asian Asparagus Salad, 154
Castor oil
  Black Salve, 75
  Castor Oil and Witch Hazel
    Makeup Remover, 48
  Essential Earache Rub, 76
Cayenne pepper
  Curried Root Vegetable
    Soup, 142
  Sweet and Spicy Barbecue
    Sauce, 125
Celeriac root
  Roasted Maple Celeriac, 131
Celery
  Chicken-Broccoli Soup, 141
  Citrus Joint Juice, 67
  Curried Root Vegetable
    Soup, 142
  Homemade Beef Stock, 138
  Homemade Chicken Stock, 139
  Mustard Chicken Salad, 146
  Roasted Tomato Soup, 144
  Spicy Sloppy Joes, 175
Cellulite, 26
Chamomile Conditioning Rinse, 60

Chamomile tea bags
  Chamomile Conditioning
    Rinse, 60
  Hair-Shining Tea and Sea
    Spray, 61
  Parched Skin Peppermint
    Spray, 56
Cheddar cheese
  Bacon and Cheddar Breakfast
    Scones, 113
Cheese. *See* Cheddar cheese;
    Feta cheese; Goat cheese;
    Parmesan cheese
Cherry-Apple Cider Nectar, 66
Cherry juice
  Cherry-Apple Cider Nectar, 66
Cherry tomatoes
  Greek Couscous Salad, 149
  Grilled Vegetable Pasta
    Salad, 150
  Sun-Dried Tomato
    Vinaigrette, 128
  Watermelon-Tomato Salad, 155
Chia seeds
  Mango-Ginger Smoothie, 97
Chicken
  Chicken-Broccoli Soup, 141
  Chicken Pot Pie, 165–166
  Chinese Chicken Lettuce
    Wraps, 169
  Homemade Chicken Stock, 139
  Honey Tomato Chicken
    Drumsticks, 168
  Hot and Sour Soup, 140
  Mustard Chicken Salad, 146
Chicken broth
  Bone Broth Sipper, 84
  Chicken-Broccoli Soup, 141
  Chicken Pot Pie, 165–166
  Eggs Poached in Ratatouille, 118
  Hot and Sour Soup, 140
  Maple Cider Pork Chops, 174
  Oktoberfest Stew, 145
  Roasted Tomato Soup, 144
Chili Dry Rub Pork Ribs, 172–173
Chili paste
  Asian Asparagus Salad, 154
Chili powder
  Chili Dry Rub Pork Ribs,
    172–173

Cocoa-Chili Bundt Cake, 184
Spicy Sloppy Joes, 175
Sweet and Spicy Barbecue
  Sauce, 125
Chinese Chicken Lettuce
  Wraps, 169
Chives
  Creamy Scrambled Eggs, 119
Chocolate chips
  Chocolate Layer Cake, 196–197
  Chocolate-Peanut Butter
    Cookies, 186–187
Chocolate Layer Cake, 196–197
Chocolate Mineral Smoothie, 81
Chocolate-Peanut Butter
  Cookies, 186–187
Cilantro
  Asian Asparagus Salad, 154
  Curried Root Vegetable
    Soup, 142
  Flank Steak with Citrus
    Marinade, 176
  Gazpacho Smoothie, 102
  Spiced Carrot Salad, 147
  Tahini Curry Noodle Bowl,
    158–159
  Watermelon-Tomato Salad, 155
  Wild Rice Bowl, 160
Cinnamon
  Apple Pie Drink, 92
  Blueberry Muffins, 110
  Cinnamon Apple Breakfast
    Cake, 111
  Creamy Peach Smoothie, 106
  Dark Chocolate Pancakes, 115
  Elderberry Shrub, 70
  Fennel Tea, 83
  Four Thieves Vinegar, 71
  Honey-Lemon Tea, 93
  Licorice Root Gargle, 85
  Pear Green Smoothie, 101
  Pumpkin Pie Enzyme Mask, 45
Citrus Cypress Spray, 58
Citrus Joint Juice, 67
Citrus Refresher, 91
Clean Fifteen, 200
Cleopatra, 18–19
Clove essential oil
  Plantain Poultice, 74
  Warm Mint Compress, 80

Cloves
  Apple Pie Drink, 92
  Banana-Berry Smoothie, 105
  Elderberry Shrub, 70
  Four Thieves Vinegar, 71
  Tomato Ketchup, 124
  Traditional Sauerbraten, 177
Club soda
  Lime-Cider Soda, 94
Cocoa powder
  Chocolate Layer Cake, 196–197
  Chocolate Mineral Smoothie, 81
  Cocoa-Chili Bundt Cake, 184
  Dark Chocolate Pancakes, 115
Coconut
  Tropical Cider Smoothie, 98
Coconut milk
  Tahini Curry Noodle Bowl,
    158–159
  Tropical Cider Smoothie, 98
Coconut oil
  Black Salve, 75
  Blueberry Muffin, 110
  Cocoa-Chili Bundt Cake, 184
  Cracked Heel Salve with Rice, 51
  Dark Chocolate Pancakes, 115
  Exfoliating Lemon-Sugar Scalp
    Scrub, 47
  Lavender-Coconut Hair Mask, 61
  Orange-Coconut Constipation
    Chews, 73
Cold and flu
  Elderberry Shrub, 70
  Fire Cider, 69
  Four Thieves Vinegar, 71
  Vinegar Vapor for Stuffy
    Sinuses, 68
Columbus, Christopher, 22
Condiments
  Berry Vinaigrette, 126
  Green Goddess Dressing, 129
  Herb-Flower Vinegar, 130
  Roasted Maple Celeriac, 131
  Sun-Dried Tomato
    Vinaigrette, 128
  Sweet and Spicy Barbecue
    Sauce, 125
  Tomato Ketchup, 124
Congestion, 26

Constipation
    Orange-Coconut Constipation
      Chews, 73
    Psyllium Solution, 72
    Tender Tummy Rub, 73
Conversion tables, 199
Coriander
    Spiced Carrot Salad, 147
    Tahini Curry Noodle
      Bowl, 158–159
Corn
    Maple Salmon Packets with
      Asian Vegetables, 167
Cotton cloth, 34
Couscous, Greek, Salad, 149
Cracked Heel Salve with Rice, 51
Cranberries
    Fennel-Jicama Salad, 152
    Wild Rice Bowl, 160
Creamy Mashed Potatoes, 134
Creamy Peach Smoothie, 106
Creamy Scrambled Eggs, 119
Cucumbers. See also English
    cucumbers
    Cucumber-Lemon Cleanser, 63
Culture, apple cider vinegar
    in, 18–19
Cumin
    Chili Dry Rub Pork
      Ribs, 172–173
    Spiced Carrot Salad, 147
    Tahini Curry Noodle
      Bowl, 158–159
Currants
    Irish Bannock, 112
Curried Root Vegetable Soup, 142
Cuts, stings, bites, and scrapes
    Black Salve, 75
    Plantain Poultice, 74
Cypress essential oil
    Citrus Cypress Spray, 58

D

Dandruff, 26
    Exfoliating Lemon-Sugar Scalp
      Scrub, 47
    Nettle and Tea Tree Rinse, 46
Dark Chocolate Pancakes, 115

Desserts
    Apple Cider Vinegar Meringues
      with Raspberries, 180–181
    Apple Cider Vinegar Pie,
      190–191
    Apple Cinnamon Scones, 183
    Blueberry Cobbler, 194–195
    Chocolate Layer Cake, 196–197
    Chocolate-Peanut Butter
      Cookies, 186–187
    Cocoa-Chili Bundt Cake, 184
    Lemon Pudding Cake, 193
    Tangy Panna Cotta with
      Strawberries, 182
    Tarte Tatin, 188–189
Detox cleansing, 26
Dijon mustard
    Chili Dry Rub Pork
      Ribs, 172–173
    Honey Tomato Chicken
      Drumsticks, 168
    Mustard Chicken Salad, 146
    Potato Salad with Hot Bacon
      Dressing, 151
    Spicy Sloppy Joes, 175
Dill seed
    Garlic Dill Pickles, 133
Dirty Dozen, 200
Double Almond Muffins, 114
Drinks and smoothies
    Almond-Berry Smoothie, 96
    Apple Pie Drink, 92
    Avocado-Herb Smoothie, 104
    Banana-Berry Smoothie, 105
    Bright Carrot Smoothie, 103
    Citrus Refresher, 91
    Creamy Peach Smoothie, 106
    Gazpacho Smoothie, 102
    Honey-Lemon Tea, 93
    Lime-Cider Soda, 94
    Mango-Ginger Smoothie, 97
    PB and J Smoothie, 99
    Pear Green Smoothie, 101
    Raspberry Lemonade, 90
    Tropical Cider Smoothie, 98
Dry hair
    Chamomile Conditioning
      Rinse, 60

    Hair-Shining Tea and Sea
      Spray, 61
    Lavender-Coconut Hair Mask, 61
Dry skin
    Castor Oil and Witch Hazel
      Makeup Remover, 48
    Mango Skin Slougher, 49
    Rosewater and Sea Salt Body
      Spray, 49

E

Earache
    Allium Ear Dropper, 77
    Essential Earache Rub, 76
Eczema, 26
Eggplant
    Eggs Poached in Ratatouille, 118
Eggs
    Creamy Scrambled Eggs, 119
    Double Almond Muffins, 114
    Eggs Poached in Ratatouille, 118
    Flaky Biscuit and Egg
      Sandwiches, 120–121
    Golden French Toast, 116
    Hot and Sour Soup, 140
    Linguine Carbonara, 170
Egg whites
    Apple Cider Vinegar Meringues
      with Raspberries, 180–181
Elderberry Shrub, 70
English cucumbers. See also
    Cucumbers
    Banana-Berry Smoothie, 105
    Gazpacho Smoothie, 102
    Greek Couscous Salad, 149
    Watermelon-Tomato Salad, 155
Epsom salts
    Lime and Mint Salt Scrub, 50
    Rosemary–Epsom Salts
      Soak, 59
Equipment, 33–34
Escherichia coli, 23
Essential Earache Rub, 76
Ethanoic acid, 22
Eucalyptus essential oil
    Plantain Poultice, 74
Exfoliating Lemon-Sugar Scalp
    Scrub, 47

F

Farfalle pasta
  Grilled Vegetable Pasta
    Salad, 150
Fatigue, 26
Fennel essential oil
  Peppermint, Ginger, and
    Fennel Sipper, 78
  Tender Tummy Rub, 73
Fennel-Jicama Salad, 152
Fennel Tea, 83
Fermentation, 14, 17, 35
Feta cheese
  Greek Couscous Salad, 149
  Watermelon-Tomato Salad, 155
Finished ferments, 35
Fire Cider, 69
Flaky Biscuit and Egg
    Sandwiches, 120–121
Flank Steak with Citrus
    Marinade, 176
Flaxseed
  PB and J Smoothie, 99
Food, apple cider vinegar in, 19
Foot care
  Antifungal Tea Tree Nail Soak, 51
  Cracked Heel Salve with Rice, 51
  Lime and Mint Salt Scrub, 50
Four Thieves Vinegar, 71
Fruit flies, 36

G

Garlic
  Allium Ear Dropper, 77
  Asian Asparagus Salad, 154
  Bone Broth Sipper, 84
  Chicken-Broccoli Soup, 141
  Chili Dry Rub Pork
    Ribs, 172–173
  Chinese Chicken Lettuce
    Wraps, 169
  Curried Root Vegetable
    Soup, 142
  Eggs Poached in Ratatouille, 118
  Fire Cider, 69
  Flank Steak with Citrus
    Marinade, 176
  Four Thieves Vinegar, 71

Garlic Dill Pickles, 133
  Green Goddess Dressing, 129
  Herb-Marinated Halibut, 163
  Homemade Beef Stock, 138
  Homemade Chicken Stock, 139
  Honey Tomato Chicken
    Drumsticks, 168
  Linguine Carbonara, 170
  Oktoberfest Stew, 145
  Potato Salad with Hot Bacon
    Dressing, 151
  Roasted Tomato Soup, 144
  Spiced Carrot Salad, 147
  Sun-Dried Tomato
    Vinaigrette, 128
  Sweet and Spicy Barbecue
    Sauce, 125
  Wheat Berry-Stuffed
    Tomatoes, 161
  Wild Rice Bowl, 160
Garlic Dill Pickles, 133
Gazpacho Smoothie, 102
Geranium essential oil
  Cracked Heel Salve with Rice, 51
Ginger
  Asian Asparagus Salad, 154
  Avocado-Herb Smoothie, 104
  Blueberry Cobbler, 194–195
  Chinese Chicken Lettuce
    Wraps, 169
  Curried Root Vegetable
    Soup, 142
  Elderberry Shrub, 70
  Fire Cider, 69
  Flank Steak with Citrus
    Marinade, 176
  Ginger Switchel, 82
  Lime-Cider Soda, 94
  Mango-Ginger Smoothie, 97
  Maple Salmon Packets with
    Asian Vegetables, 167
  Pumpkin Pie Enzyme Mask, 45
  Roasted Maple Celeriac, 131
  Tahini Curry Noodle
    Bowl, 158–159
  Wild Rice Bowl, 160
Ginger essential oil
  Peppermint, Ginger, and
    Fennel Sipper, 78
  Tender Tummy Rub, 73

Goat cheese
  Grilled Vegetable Pasta
    Salad, 150
  Wheat Berry-Stuffed
    Tomatoes, 161
Golden French Toast, 116
Grapefruit juice
  Citrus Joint Juice, 67
Greek Couscous Salad, 149
Greek yogurt
  Creamy Peach Smoothie, 106
Green cabbage
  Oktoberfest Stew, 145
Green Goddess Dressing, 129
Green tea bags
  Parched Skin Peppermint
    Spray, 56
Grilled Vegetable Pasta Salad, 150
Ground beef
  Spicy Sloppy Joes, 175

H

Hair-Shining Tea and Sea Spray, 61
Halibut, Herb-Marinated, 163
Hand care
  Lemon-Lavender Hand Spray, 53
  Pre-Mani Nail Soak, 52
Hannibal, 18
Heartburn and indigestion, 26
  Aloe-Lemon Shooter, 79
  Peppermint, Ginger, and
    Fennel Sipper, 78
Heavy cream
  Apple Cinnamon Scones, 183
  Chocolate Layer Cake, 196–197
  Curried Root Vegetable
    Soup, 142
  Linguine Carbonara, 170
  Roasted Tomato Soup, 144
  Scallops with Bacon Cream
    Sauce, 162
  Tangy Panna Cotta with
    Strawberries, 182
Helichrysum essential oil
  Magnesium Massage Oil, 59
Herb-Flower Vinegar, 130
Herb-Marinated Halibut, 163
Hills, Margaret, 25
Hippocrates, 8, 18

History, apple cider vinegar in, 18–19
Hoisin sauce
    Chinese Chicken Lettuce Wraps, 169
Homemade apple cider vinegar, 31–38
Homemade Beef Stock, 138
Homemade Chicken Stock, 139
Honey, 32–33
    Almond-Berry Smoothie, 96
    Apple Pie Drink, 92
    Asian Asparagus Salad, 154
    Avocado-Herb Smoothie, 104
    Bright Carrot Smoothie, 103
    Chocolate Mineral Smoothie, 81
    Citrus Joint Juice, 67
    Citrus Refresher, 91
    Cracked Heel Salve with Rice, 51
    Creamy Peach Smoothie, 106
    Double Almond Muffins, 114
    Elderberry Shrub, 70
    Fennel-Jicama Salad, 152
    Fennel Tea, 83
    Fire Cider, 69
    Ginger Switchel, 82
    Green Goddess Dressing, 129
    Honey-Lemon Tea, 93
    Honey Tomato Chicken Drumsticks, 168
    Lavender-Coconut Hair Mask, 61
    Lavender-Oatmeal Soak, 57
    Licorice Root Gargle, 85
    Lime-Cider Soda, 94
    Lip-Lightening Paste, 55
    Mango Skin Slougher, 49
    Mustard Chicken Salad, 146
    Orange-Coconut Constipation Chews, 73
    PB and J Smoothie, 99
    Psyllium Solution, 72
    Raspberry Lemonade, 90
    Scallops with Bacon Cream Sauce, 162
    Spiced Carrot Salad, 147
    Sweet and Spicy Barbecue Sauce, 125
    Tomato Ketchup, 124

Horseradish
    Fire Cider, 69
Hot and Sour Soup, 140
Hot sauce
    Bone Broth Sipper, 84
    Gazpacho Smoothie, 102
Hyperpigmentation
    Aloe Vera-Turmeric Gel Facial, 54
    Applesauce and Papaya Purée Peel, 55
    Lip-Lightening Paste, 55

I
Irish Bannock, 112

J
Jalapeño chile
    Fire Cider, 69
Jellyfish stings, 26
Jicama
    Fennel-Jicama Salad, 152
    Wild Rice Bowl, 160
Johansson, Scarlett, 24
Joint pain, 26
Jojoba oil
    Lemon-Lavender Hand Spray, 53
    Magnesium Massage Oil, 59
Jones, Prudence, 19

K
Kale
    Almond-Berry Smoothie, 96
    Asian Asparagus Salad, 154
    Mango-Ginger Smoothie, 97
    Tahini Curry Noodle Bowl, 158–159
Kefir, 17
Klum, Heidi, 24
Kombucha, 17
Kvass, 17

L
Large pores, 26
Lavender
    Four Thieves Vinegar, 71
Lavender essential oil
    Black Salve, 75
    Chamomile Conditioning Rinse, 60
    Essential Earache Rub, 76
    Lavender-Coconut Hair Mask, 61
    Lavender-Oatmeal Soak, 57
    Lavender Scalp Toner, 62
    Lemon-Lavender Hand Spray, 53
    Magnesium Massage Oil, 59
    Parched Skin Peppermint Spray, 56
    Plantain Poultice, 74
    Rosewater and Sea Salt Body Spray, 49
Leeks
    Curried Root Vegetable Soup, 142
Leg cramps, 26
    Chocolate Mineral Smoothie, 81
    Warm Mint Compress, 80
Lemon essential oil
    Aloe Vera-Turmeric Gel Facial, 54
    Citrus Cypress Spray, 58
    Exfoliating Lemon-Sugar Scalp Scrub, 47
    Lemon-Lavender Hand Spray, 53
    Plantain Poultice, 74
Lemongrass essential oil
    Plantain Poultice, 74
Lemon juice
    Aloe-Lemon Shooter, 79
    Citrus Joint Juice, 67
    Cucumber-Lemon Cleanser, 63
    Exfoliating Lemon-Sugar Scalp Scrub, 47
    Fennel-Jicama Salad, 152
    Four Thieves Vinegar, 71
    Ginger Switchel, 82
    Green Goddess Dressing, 129
    Grilled Vegetable Pasta Salad, 150

Hair-Shining Tea and Sea
  Spray, 61
Herb-Marinated Halibut, 163
Honey-Lemon Tea, 93
Lemon Pudding Cake, 193
Raspberry Lemonade, 90
Vinegar Vapor for Stuffy
  Sinuses, 68
Lemon-Lavender Hand Spray, 53
Lemon Pudding Cake, 193
Lemons
  Fire Cider, 69
Lettuce
  Mustard Chicken Salad, 146
Lice, 27
Licorice Root Gargle, 85
Lime and Mint Salt Scrub, 50
Lime-Cider Soda, 94
Lime essential oil
  Lime and Mint Salt Scrub, 50
Lime juice
  Asian Asparagus Salad, 154
  Bright Carrot Smoothie, 103
  Citrus Refresher, 91
  Flank Steak with Citrus
    Marinade, 177
  Gazpacho Smoothie, 102
  Lime-Cider Soda, 94
  Mustard Chicken Salad, 146
  Wild Rice Bowl, 160
Limes
  Herb-Marinated Halibut, 163
  Linguine Carbonara, 170
Lip-Lightening Paste, 55

M

Magnesium chloride flakes
  Magnesium Massage Oil, 59
Magnesium citrate powder
  Citrus Joint Juice, 67
Magnesium Massage Oil, 59
Main Entrées
  Chicken Pot Pie, 165–166
  Chili Dry Rub Pork
    Ribs, 172–173
  Chinese Chicken Lettuce
    Wraps, 169
  Flank Steak with Citrus
    Marinade, 176

Herb-Marinated Halibut, 163
Honey Tomato Chicken
  Drumsticks, 168
Linguine Carbonara, 170
Maple Cider Pork Chops, 174
Maple Salmon Packets with
  Asian Vegetables, 167
Scallops with Bacon Cream
  Sauce, 162
Spicy Sloppy Joes, 175
Tahini Curry Noodle Bowl,
  158–159
Traditional Sauerbraten, 177
Wheat Berry-Stuffed
  Tomatoes, 161
Wild Rice Bowl, 160
Mango
  Mango-Ginger Smoothie, 97
  Mango Skin Slougher, 49
Maple Cider Pork Chops, 174
Maple Salmon Packets with Asian
  Vegetables, 167
Maple syrup
  Apple Cinnamon Scones, 183
  Bacon and Cheddar Breakfast
    Scones, 113
  Maple Cider Pork Chops, 174
  Maple Salmon Packets with
    Asian Vegetables, 167
  Roasted Maple Celeriac, 131
Marc Antony, 18–19
Medicine, apple cider vinegar
  in, 18
Milk. *See also* Almond milk;
  Coconut milk
  Bacon and Cheddar Breakfast
    Scones, 113
  Banana-Berry Smoothie, 105
  Blueberry Muffins, 110
  Cinnamon Apple Breakfast
    Cake, 111
  Creamy Mashed Potatoes, 134
  Creamy Scrambled Eggs, 119
  Dark Chocolate Pancakes, 115
  Flaky Biscuit and Egg
    Sandwiches, 120–121
  Golden French Toast, 116
  Irish Bannock, 112
  Tangy Panna Cotta with
    Strawberries, 182

Mint
  Avocado-Herb Smoothie, 104
  Four Thieves Vinegar, 71
  Lime-Cider Soda, 94
  Vinegar Vapor for Stuffy
    Sinuses, 68
  Watermelon-Tomato Salad, 155
Molasses
  Spicy Sloppy Joes, 175
  Sweet and Spicy Barbecue
    Sauce, 125
Mold, 36
Mouthwash, 25
Muffins
  Blueberry Muffins, 110
  Double Almond Muffins, 114
Mushrooms
  Grilled Vegetable Pasta
    Salad, 150
  Hot and Sour Soup, 140
  Scallops with Bacon Cream
    Sauce, 162
Mustard. *See* Dijon mustard
Mustard Chicken Salad, 146

N

Napa cabbage
  Wild Rice Bowl, 160
Napoleon, 19
Nausea and morning sickness, 25
  Fennel Tea, 83
  Ginger Switchel, 82
Nettle and Tea Tree Rinse, 46
Nursing, apple cider vinegar
  and, 24
Nutmeg
  Lime-Cider Soda, 94
  Pear Green Smoothie, 101
  Pumpkin Pie Enzyme Mask, 45

O

Oats
  Apple Cinnamon Scones, 183
  Lavender-Oatmeal Soak, 57
  Mango Skin Slougher, 49
"Off" flavors, 37

Oily hair
Cucumber-Lemon Cleanser, 63
Lavender Scalp Toner, 62
Oktoberfest Stew, 145
Olive oil
Berry Vinaigrette, 126
Chicken-Broccoli Soup, 141
Greek Couscous Salad, 149
Green Goddess Dressing, 129
Grilled Vegetable Pasta Salad,
150
Herb-Marinated Halibut, 163
Honey Tomato Chicken
Drumsticks, 168
Lemon-Lavender Hand Spray, 53
Lime and Mint Salt Scrub, 50
Maple Cider Pork Chops, 174
Mustard Chicken Salad, 146
Oktoberfest Stew, 145
Pre-Mani Nail Soak, 52
Roasted Maple Celeriac, 131
Roasted Tomato Soup, 144
Spiced Carrot Salad, 147
Sun-Dried Tomato
Vinaigrette, 128
Sweet and Spicy Barbecue
Sauce, 125
Tahini Curry Noodle
Bowl, 158–159
Tender Tummy Rub, 73
Traditional Sauerbraten, 177
Watermelon-Tomato Salad, 155
Wild Rice Bowl, 160
Onion powder
Chili Dry Rub Pork Ribs,
172–173
Sweet and Spicy Barbecue
Sauce, 125
Onions. See also Red onions
Allium Ear Dropper, 77
Bavarian Braised Red
Cabbage, 135
Chicken-Broccoli Soup, 141
Chicken Pot Pie, 165–166
Curried Root Vegetable
Soup, 142
Eggs Poached in Ratatouille, 118
Fire Cider, 69
Homemade Beef Stock, 138

Homemade Chicken Stock, 139
Oktoberfest Stew, 145
Roasted Tomato Soup, 144
Spicy Sloppy Joes, 175
Traditional Sauerbraten, 177
Wheat Berry-Stuffed
Tomatoes, 161
Orange-Coconut Constipation
Chews, 73
Orange essential oil
Aloe Vera-Turmeric Gel
Facial, 54
Pumpkin Pie Enzyme Mask, 45
Orange juice
Citrus Joint Juice, 67
Citrus Refresher, 91
Flank Steak with Citrus
Marinade, 177
Mustard Chicken Salad, 146
Orange-Coconut Constipation
Chews, 73
Oranges
Fire Cider, 69
Oregano
Eggs Poached in Ratatouille, 118
Greek Couscous Salad, 149
Herb-Marinated Halibut, 163
Roasted Tomato Soup, 144
Spicy Sloppy Joes, 175
Sun-Dried Tomato
Vinaigrette, 128
Organic herb flowers
Herb-Flower Vinegar, 130

P

Papaya
Applesauce and Papaya Purée
Peel, 55
Parched Skin Peppermint
Spray, 56
Parmesan cheese
Linguine Carbonara, 170
Parsley
Avocado-Herb Smoothie, 104
Chicken-Broccoli Soup, 141
Green Goddess Dressing, 129
Linguine Carbonara, 170
Mustard Chicken Salad, 146
Oktoberfest Stew, 145

Potato Salad with Hot Bacon
Dressing, 151
Spiced Carrot Salad, 147
Wheat Berry-Stuffed
Tomatoes, 161
Parsnips
Curried Root Vegetable
Soup, 142
PB and J Smoothie, 99
Peaches
Creamy Peach Smoothie, 106
Peanut butter
PB and J Smoothie, 99
Peanut butter chips
Chocolate-Peanut Butter
Cookies, 186–187
Pear Green Smoothie, 101
Pears
Bright Carrot Smoothie, 103
Pear Green Smoothie, 101
Peas. See also Snow peas
Chicken Pot Pie, 165–166
Pectin, 29, 32
Peppercorns
Fire Cider, 69
Garlic Dill Pickles, 133
Homemade Beef Stock, 138
Homemade Chicken Stock, 139
Peppermint essential oil
Lime and Mint Salt Scrub, 50
Parched Skin Peppermint
Spray, 56
Peppermint, Ginger, and
Fennel Sipper, 78
Warm Mint Compress, 80
Phytochemicals, 23
Pickling cucumbers
Garlic Dill Pickles, 133
Pickling salt
Garlic Dill Pickles, 133
Pineapple
Tropical Cider Smoothie, 98
Pistachios
Wild Rice Bowl, 160
Plantain Poultice, 74
Polyphenols, 23
Pork
Chili Dry Rub Pork
Ribs, 172–173
Maple Cider Pork Chops, 174

Potatoes
    Chicken Pot Pie, 165–166
    Creamy Mashed Potatoes, 134
    Oktoberfest Stew, 145
    Potato Salad with Hot Bacon
      Dressing, 151
Prebiotics, 29
Pregnancy, apple cider vinegar
    and, 24
Pre-Mani Nail Soak, 52
Prescription medicine interac-
    tions, 24
Probiotics, 29
Psoriasis, 27
Psyllium Solution, 72
Puff pastry
    Tarte Tatin, 188–189
Pumpkin Pie Enzyme Mask, 45
Pumpkin seeds
    Curried Root Vegetable
      Soup, 142

R

Radishes
    Fennel-Jicama Salad, 152
Raisins
    Irish Bannock, 112
    Spiced Carrot Salad, 147
Rashes, 27
Raspberries
    Almond-Berry Smoothie, 96
    Apple Cider Vinegar Meringues
      with Raspberries, 180–181
    Berry Vinaigrette, 126
    Lip-Lightening Paste, 55
    Raspberry Lemonade, 90
Red bell peppers
    Chinese Chicken Lettuce
      Wraps, 169
    Eggs Poached in Ratatouille, 118
    Greek Couscous Salad, 149
    Grilled Vegetable Pasta
      Salad, 150
    Hot and Sour Soup, 140
    Mustard Chicken Salad, 146
    Spicy Sloppy Joes, 175
    Tahini Curry Noodle
      Bowl, 158–159
    Wild Rice Bowl, 160

Red cabbage
    Bavarian Braised Red
      Cabbage, 135
Red onions
    Greek Couscous Salad, 149
    Grilled Vegetable Pasta
      Salad, 150
Resources, 201
Rice, Cracked Heel Salve with, 51
Rice noodles
    Tahini Curry Noodle
      Bowl, 158–159
Ringworm, 27
Roasted Maple Celeriac, 131
Roasted Tomato Soup, 144
Rosemary
    Fire Cider, 69
    Four Thieves Vinegar, 71
Rosemary essential oil
    Hair-Shining Tea and Sea
      Spray, 61
    Plantain Poultice, 74
    Rosemary–Epsom Salts
      Soak, 59
Rosewater and Sea Salt Body
    Spray, 49
Rubbing alcohol
    Allium Ear Dropper, 77
Ruby red grapefruit juice
    Citrus Refresher, 91

S

Sage
    Four Thieves Vinegar, 71
Salads
    Asian Asparagus Salad, 154
    Fennel-Jicama Salad, 152
    Greek Couscous Salad, 149
    Grilled Vegetable Pasta
      Salad, 150
    Mustard Chicken Salad, 146
    Potato Salad with Hot Bacon
      Dressing, 151
    Spiced Carrot Salad, 147
    Watermelon-Tomato Salad, 155
Salmon, Maple, Packets with
    Asian Vegetables, 167
Sausage
    Oktoberfest Stew, 145

Scallions
    Asian Asparagus Salad, 154
    Chinese Chicken Lettuce
      Wraps, 169
    Fennel-Jicama Salad, 152
    Greek Couscous Salad, 149
    Green Goddess Dressing, 129
    Hot and Sour Soup, 140
    Maple Salmon Packets with
      Asian Vegetables, 167
    Mustard Chicken Salad, 146
    Potato Salad with Hot Bacon
      Dressing, 151
    Watermelon-Tomato Salad, 155
    Wild Rice Bowl, 160
Scallops with Bacon Cream
    Sauce, 162
Scarring, 27
SCOBY, 17
Scones
    Apple Cinnamon Scones, 183
    Bacon and Cheddar Breakfast
      Scones, 113
Seafood
    Herb-Marinated Halibut, 163
    Maple Salmon Packets with
      Asian Vegetables, 167
    Scallops with Bacon Cream
      Sauce, 162
Sea salt
    Chocolate Mineral Smoothie, 81
    Green Goddess Dressing, 129
    Licorice Root Gargle, 85
    Orange-Coconut Constipation
      Chews, 73
    Parched Skin Peppermint
      Spray, 56
Sesame oil
    Asian Asparagus Salad, 154
Shampoo buildup, 27
Sides
    Bavarian Braised Red
      Cabbage, 135
    Creamy Mashed Potatoes, 134
    Garlic Dill Pickles, 133
    Roasted Maple Celeriac, 131
Slippery elm powder
    Orange-Coconut Constipation
      Chews, 73

Snow peas
    Chinese Chicken Lettuce
        Wraps, 169
    Tahini Curry Noodle
        Bowl, 158–159
Sore throat, 27
    Bone Broth Sipper, 84
    Licorice Root Gargle, 85
Soups
    Chicken-Broccoli Soup, 141
    Curried Root Vegetable
        Soup, 142
    Homemade Beef Stock, 138
    Homemade Chicken Stock, 139
    Hot and Sour Soup, 140
    Oktoberfest Stew, 145
    Roasted Tomato Soup, 144
Soy sauce
    Chinese Chicken Lettuce
        Wraps, 169
    Flank Steak with Citrus
        Marinade, 177
Spiced Carrot Salad, 147
Spicy Sloppy Joes, 175
Spinach
    Avocado-Herb Smoothie, 104
    Chocolate Mineral Smoothie, 81
    Pear Green Smoothie, 101
Sterilization, 35
Stomach, apple cider vinegar
    and, 24
Storage bottles, 34
Strainer, 34
Strawberries
    Almond-Berry Smoothie, 96
    Banana-Berry Smoothie, 105
    Berry Vinaigrette, 126
    Mango-Ginger Smoothie, 97
    PB and J Smoothie, 99
    Tangy Panna Cotta with
        Strawberries, 182
Sucanat
    Exfoliating Lemon-Sugar Scalp
        Scrub, 47
Sugar, 32–33
Sunburn, 27
    Lavender-Oatmeal Soak, 57
    Parched Skin Peppermint
        Spray, 56

Sun-dried tomatoes
    Sun-Dried Tomato
        Vinaigrette, 128
Sunflower seeds
    Pear Green Smoothie, 101
Sung Tse, 18
Sunlight, in fermenting
    environment, 35
Sun spots, 27
Sweet almond oil
    Hair-Shining Tea and Sea
        Spray, 61
    Lip-Lightening Paste, 55
    Parched Skin Peppermint
        Spray, 56
Sweet and Spicy Barbecue
    Sauce, 125

T

Tahini Curry Noodle
    Bowl, 158–159
Tamari sauce
    Maple Salmon Packets with
        Asian Vegetables, 167
Tangy Panna Cotta with
    Strawberries, 182
Tarragon
    Chicken Pot Pie, 165–166
Tarte Tatin, 188–189
Tea tree essential oil
    Antifungal Tea Tree Nail Soak, 51
    Black Salve, 75
    Essential Earache Rub, 76
    Nettle and Tea Tree Rinse, 46
    Plantain Poultice, 74
Teeth, apple cider vinegar and, 24
Temperature in fermenting
    environment, 35
Tender Tummy Rub, 73
Thinning hair, 27
Thyme
    Bright Carrot Smoothie, 103
    Chicken-Broccoli Soup, 141
    Chicken Pot Pie, 165–166
    Fire Cider, 69
    Four Thieves Vinegar, 71
    Herb-Marinated Halibut, 163

Homemade Chicken Stock, 139
    Scallops with Bacon Cream
        Sauce, 162
Thyme essential oil
    Plantain Poultice, 74
Tomatoes. *See also* Cherry toma-
    toes; Sun-dried tomatoes
    Eggs Poached in Ratatouille, 118
    Gazpacho Smoothie, 102
    Roasted Tomato Soup, 144
    Wheat Berry-Stuffed
        Tomatoes, 161
Tomato juice
    Gazpacho Smoothie, 102
Tomato Ketchup, 124
Tomato paste
    Honey Tomato Chicken
        Drumsticks, 168
    Spicy Sloppy Joes, 175
    Sweet and Spicy Barbecue
        Sauce, 125
    Tomato Ketchup, 124
Traditional Sauerbraten, 177
Tropical Cider Smoothie, 98
Troubleshooting guide, 36–37
Turmeric
    Aloe Vera-Turmeric Gel
        Facial, 54
    Fire Cider, 69
    Tahini Curry Noodle
        Bowl, 158–159

V

Varicose veins, 27
    Citrus Cypress Spray, 58
    Magnesium Massage Oil, 59
    Rosemary-Epsom Salts Soak, 59
Vegetable broth
    Bavarian Braised Red
        Cabbage, 135
    Curried Root Vegetable
        Soup, 142
Vinegar Vapor for Stuffy
    Sinuses, 68
Vitamin E oil
    Aloe Vera-Turmeric Gel
        Facial, 54
    Lemon-Lavender Hand Spray, 53

Magnesium Massage Oil, 59
Pumpkin Pie Enzyme Mask, 45

W

Warm Mint Compress, 80
Warts, 27
Water, 33
Watermelon-Tomato Salad, 155
Weak hair, 27
Weight gain, 27
Wheat Berry-Stuffed
    Tomatoes, 161
White wine
    Linguine Carbonara, 170
Wild Rice Bowl, 160
Wintergreen essential oil
    Lime and Mint Salt Scrub, 50
    Warm Mint Compress, 80
Witch hazel
    Castor Oil and Witch Hazel
        Makeup Remover, 48
    Citrus Cypress Spray, 58
Worcestershire sauce
    Honey Tomato Chicken
        Drumsticks, 168

Y

Yellow bell peppers
    Wheat Berry-Stuffed
        Tomatoes, 161
Yellow teeth, 27
Yogurt. *See also* Greek yogurt
    Chocolate Mineral Smoothie, 81

Z

Zucchini
    Eggs Poached in Ratatouille, 118
    Grilled Vegetable Pasta
        Salad, 150

ABOUT THE AUTHOR

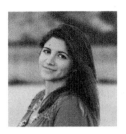 **MADELINE GIVEN** is a certified holistic nutrition consultant and health educator. She works predominantly with women, helping them find the freedom of health in their ever-changing bodies. For wellness wisdom and real food recipes, visit her blog, MadelineNutrition.com. You can also find her online at @madelinenutrition on Instagram and facebook.com/madelinenutrition. She currently lives in Santa Barbara, California, with her husband.